Praise for *Annette: A Nurse's Story*

Immediately engaging, instantly interesting, Annette's story is one of her own awakening, unfolding self-awareness, intellectual growth, and ultimately the discovery of her authentic passion. Her true passion is to innovatively change forever the education of nurses by advancing the notion of higher education for nurses — university-based education through scholarship focusing on what nurses know, not hospital training based on apprenticeship focusing on what nurses do. She proposes a curriculum that moves nursing education well beyond the confining walls of the hospital in which an entrenched, industrialized, mechanized, reductionist model of healthcare existed in America just prior to the turn of the twentieth century.

Annette emerges as a disruptive leader advocating for the professionalization of nursing on a par with medicine and dentistry. To accomplish this, she proposes a scholastic education for nurses which incorporates the basic and applied sciences, including biology, chemistry, and anatomy and physiology as well as mathematics, cultural and social studies, and religion. This new model of nursing education requires a curriculum that prepares graduates for knowledge-based nursing practice that can occur in environs well beyond the confines of the hospital. In fact, Annette envisions knowledge-based nursing practice that can occur wherever people exist — homes, schools, industry, larger communities, and yes, even hospitals.

With faith and hope as her credo, Annette is driven by her curiosity, evolving sense of purpose, and growing passion to imagine a society in which health is conceptualized, not as the mere absence of disease. Our heroine sees a newly emerging and evolving culture of health focusing on health maintenance and disease prevention before it occurs rather than the mere treatment of disease after it is diagnosed. To achieve this newfound culture of health, there must be a careful differentiation between the practice of medicine, the diagnosis, treatment and management of disease and the practice of nursing, the use of education as an essential tool to restore and maintain health.

Annette's vision and politic are of evolving social change and creating an enduring legacy of improved healthcare and healthcare education—all requiring a tremendous shift in the paradigm of health, healthcare, and the education of health professionals. All of this occurring within the context of the nineteenth century's overwhelming patriarchy and society's profound public health challenges compounded by poverty, overcrowding, and disease, both endemic and epidemic.

Annette's story offers a commentary on power—"information is power," "organization is power," and "power is driven by action." It is also a treatise on the vision-driven leadership of highly intelligent, politically aware women acting as activist agents of change to address the complex social challenges confronting the women and society of Annette's time—women's suffrage, women's access to education, the availability and use of birth control education and methods, women's fundamental right to own property, and the prohibition of alcohol.

Annette's enlightening journey takes her from posh parlors filled with activist academics and rich socialites in the Back Bay neighborhood of Boston to the poorest overcrowded squalid tenements of Manhattan's Lower East Side. Along the way, Annette develops an in-depth understanding of power and politics. She learns that the art of politics is relationship building. She gains insight into the education and licensure of nurses and understands the dynamic interplay of laws governing both. If Annette's vision had been brought to fruition more than 100 years ago, perhaps the currently existing and enduring disconnect between collegiate nurse education and nurse licensure could have been avoided long ago.

Ward masterfully demonstrates the true art of historical fiction through storytelling that takes place at the intersection of that which is real and documented and that which is imagined and can never be truly known. She achieves this through an accurate reporting of historical facts, chronological events, and people while artfully exploring the imagined internal thoughts, conversations, and feelings of those who actually lived these events—all within the context of their own time and place. Ward accomplishes this feat through her rich, one could even say delicious, integration of descriptions of dress, environs, contemporary thought, social mores, and even the food of the 1890s.

Ward's cast of players help bring Annette's story to life and have much to teach about the human condition—their idiosyncrasies, their personal desires and motivations, their value and use of humor, and even their own private affairs of the heart. Through her creative integrative weaving of fact and fiction, Ward tells Annette's story. It is the story of a history that should have been and almost was.

David Anthony (Tony) Forrester, Ph.D., R.N., FAAN, ANEF
Professor Emeritus, School of Nursing, Rutgers University

Annette Fiske's imagined nursing story is one of radicalized intellect, tenacious vision, and political determination. Born in 1873 in Boston and educated in the classics, she is determined to forge equitable education and health care systems in late nineteenth-century America. Frances Ward compellingly tells the story of Annette, from her graduation with honors in Radcliffe College's first class awarded academic degrees in 1894 to her immersion in controversial movements — suffrage, education, hospitals, science, and nurse training — each invigorated by key leaders of the era.

Intrigued with contributions made by nurses to the public, Annette entered the Waltham Hospital Training School for Nurses, graduating in 1898. This was a transformative experience for Annette, leading her to claim that she had never really lived until she became a nurse. Annette holds President Charles W. Eliot to his inaugural promise that Harvard University would offer diverse curricula, that "we would have them all, and at their best." Under Eliot's complex scheme to achieve that goal, Annette spirits physician Alfred Worcester and a small, dedicated crew to work toward the establishment of Harvard's School of Nursing in 1900.

Herself a nursing administrator, historian, and memoirist, Ward chronicles the ferocious backlash of nurse leaders to Eliot's plan, who intended to secure the hospital as the sole place to train nurses under physician domination within an oppressive apprenticeship ethos. Despite the rapidly advancing movement to hospitalize America within a disease management orientation framed by the successes of sanitary science, Eliot and Annette covertly move America on an alternate path of higher education for nurses, using gritty political strategies and tactics to defeat diverse threats along their journey.

Once operational, the Harvard University School of Nursing quickly reforms the country's health model to one of health promotion and disease prevention, eventually laying the foundation for a national system of free comprehensive health services, a system promoting improved national health outcomes.

Within an American healthcare system that too often fails those most in need of high-quality care, Ward's novel provides an alternative vision of what could have been. And, perhaps, what might yet be so. It is a must read for all those concerned about the health disparities created within our healthcare system. It is a call to action for the nursing profession, which collectively has the wisdom and power to lead us to the healthcare model so beautifully presented in this novel.

Rhonda Maneval, D.Ed., RN, ANEF, FAAN
Professor of Nursing, Interim Provost and Dean
Carlow University

Annette: A Nurse's Story

Frances Ward

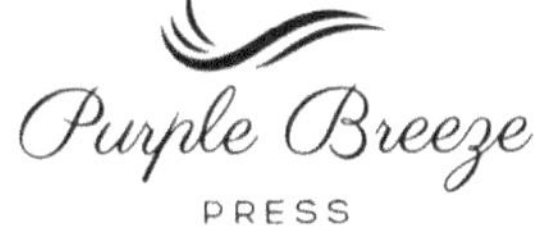

Purple Breeze
PRESS

ALSO BY FRANCES WARD

History:

On Duty: Power, Politics, and the History of Nursing in New Jersey

Memoir:

The Door of Last Resort: Memoirs of a Nurse Practitioner

Novel:

Emily in War

Purple Breeze Press, LLC

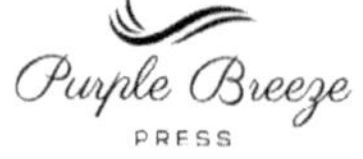

purplebreezepress.com

Annette: A Nurse's Story

Annette: A Nurse's Story is a work of historical fiction. Apart from well-known actual people and events that feature in the narrative, all characters and incidences are imagined products of the author and are used fictitiously. No content of the novel is to be understood as real.

Library of Congress Cataloguing in Publication Data

Names: Ward, Frances, author

Title: *Annette: A Nurse's Story* / Frances ward

Description: First edition. | Purple Breeze Press, 2024

Library of Congress Control Number: 2024901000

ISBN Paperback: 9798876964151

Book designed and copy edited by Meg Vezzu / megvezzu.com

Dedication

In this book, I celebrate the nurse faculty, staff, and graduates of the University of Medicine and Dentistry of New Jersey School of Nursing (since 2013, part of Rutgers-The State University of New Jersey) for their participation in a school built purposely as an anomaly.

This book is dedicated to my daughter, Sarah Ann, my nurse.

Contents

CBS News, 1975

"**M**other was a revolutionary."

With silver-gray hair swept into a large floral claw clip, Elizabeth, at seventy-three, closely resembled her mother, Annette. Her green eyes focused keenly on Daniel Schorr's face as she leaned in, drawing the attention of the Columbia Broadcasting System correspondent.

"Mr. Schorr," Elizabeth spoke so he would listen carefully, "Annette was more than a dean of nursing. She was a scholar of classical languages and literature. She was the bravest woman I ever knew."

Quizzical about the unexpected direction that his interview with Elizabeth Byrne had taken, Daniel Schorr laid his tape recorder on the desk, hastily gesturing a request for details as he checked the placement of his audiotape. The woman before him was daughter of Annette Fiske Byrne, the founding dean of Harvard University's School of Nursing. In health care, the family was American royalty.

A correspondent for CBS News since 1953, Schorr's assignment was to illuminate the life of the mother. This year, 1975, marked the seventy-fifth anniversary of the founding of Harvard's School of Nursing, the iconic institution that had rejected the hospitalization of America by shifting focus from disease to health. In one bold move, Harvard had changed the rules. Within decades, the country had shifted from physician dominance to patient self-responsibility. Across political parties and geographic regions, every American knew that theirs was the best health care system in the world.

Schorr saw himself as an international reporter of major world events, having won Emmy awards in 1972, 1973, and 1974 for outstanding achievement within regularly scheduled news programs. He enjoyed reporting on politics, even provoking the anger of Richard Nixon, with his name heading the President's Enemies List.

This is a dull assignment, Schorr mused. Only one year after my third Emmy award, am I now considered past my prime? Junior reporters were now working the major world stories, and here he was, left to record memories. Had he now moved from being a journalist to a documentarian? The thought was jarring, and he pushed it from his mind, determined to finish as quickly as possible.

In the refurbished library in Fay House, the building on Garden Street in Cambridge that had housed the Society for the Collegiate Instruction of Women founded in 1882, Schorr fidgeted with the elaborately curled hand rests of his Toscano armchair. Meeting Elizabeth's gaze, he motioned for her to continue. It was 9 am. Given time constraints, he hoped the interview would pass quickly.

Yes, Elizabeth thought, Daniel is very impatient. She wondered if he had prepared for this interview. Did he appreciate that the current universal health system had stopped forces that would squash families? The crushing hospitalization of America that had begun to emerge in the late nineteenth century? The rapacious health insurance industry lurking in the shadows, that intended to play a key role in determining patient treatments? Drug costs so high that patients would have to choose between medicine or food? Had this reporter taken the time to understand the events of 1892 to 1898 and her mother's role in them? Or was he, rather, pining for a posting to Vietnam or Saudi Arabia?

Balancing Schorr's impatience against her mother's vision and accomplishments, Elizabeth was comfortable in her role as interviewee, able to set aside his lack of interest, and to tell her mother's bold, American story. He was only the clerk. She was keeper of the story.

Softly, she continued. "I am named after my mother's aunt, Elizabeth Ellen Sedgwick, whose grandfather was a general during the American Revolution. In post-Civil War America, Charles William Eliot challenged Harvard University to radically transform education, to offer diverse curricula. As he said in his presidential inaugural address, "we would have them all, and at their best." Education—in fields as different as the sciences and arts—would propel the United States as a world leader.

"My mother," Elizabeth noted, "agreed with President Eliot."

"Few, however," Elizabeth said slowly for emphasis, "agreed with either Annette or Charles. In the late nineteenth century, women, considered property of their husbands, could not attend colleges or universities.

They could not vote. They were not employed. This you know."

"What you do not know," she added, "is that Mother was determined to hold Eliot to his inaugural promise: she would have them all. That was her mantra. She viewed education as the springboard for change, critically needed in health care."

"Daniel, to understand Annette and appreciate her accomplishments," Elizabeth's gaze bore into his eyes, "you must recognize the complex landscape framing her war—a war in which she asserted nursing an academic discipline, a profession directly responsible for maintaining, or restoring, health, for both individuals and the public."

Clicking his recorder on, Schorr moved a curl of gray hair off his black-rimmed glasses resting on slightly reddened cheeks and settled into his large armchair. There might be, he realized, a story here worth telling.

"As we continue, Elizabeth," suggested Schorr, with less urgency in his voice than previously, "please remind me of your mother's relationship with the National Institutes of Health and the Centers for Health Promotion. I understand that both were originally designed quite differently than their final forms. What was Annette's role in the establishment of these entities?"

"Yes, Annette, her colleague Alfred Worcester, and President Eliot played essential roles in the design of both the NIH and the CHP. In fact, they averted the creation of a dystopian health care system." Elizabeth sipped the tea that had been served to them at the beginning of the interview.

"Elizabeth, say more." Schorr stopped looking at his watch. "I can stay longer than one hour, if you can also."

Elizabeth smiled and said that she could.

Rage

"Never again!"

Enraged, Annette dropped her white bonnet and matching riding gloves, saturated with rain and streaked with mud, onto a chair facing Elizabeth Agassiz's large oak desk. As Annette scowled silently at Elizabeth, the older woman's head remained fixed on her writing paper, her dip pen tapping the tip against the rim of the inkwell.

"Annette, should you not be in class?"

Shifting attention momentarily to Annette, the president of the Society for the Collegiate Instruction of Women met the student's gaze without lifting her head. Elizabeth, at seventy-two, remained a formidable woman. With long gray hair parted in the middle and wrapped into a tight bun at the nape of her neck, she was stately — almost statuesque, seemingly impenetrable. Elizabeth had an institutional reputation to consider, and this girl's appearance — with wet torn dress, disheveled hair, and scratches on her arms — offended her. In Elizabeth's plan, the society, colloquially called the Harvard Annex, would be the forerunner of a sister institution to Harvard University for women. She waited for the damp girl to speak.

"I *want* to be in class!"

Still seething, Annette described her bicycle route from her home at 1564 Massachusetts Avenue to Fay House on Garden Street. Usually a half-mile, fifteen-minute ride, today the trip was longer, given heavy rain, muddy streets, and downed tree branches.

"As you can see, I fell off my bike. My Victoria Model bicycle is my independence, my freedom. It is now damaged, my outfit ruined. Had I taken a shortcut through Harvard Yard, I might not have fallen. The Yard has even paths, with less risk of falling."

Beyond breathless, Annette was spent. Tossing her wet bonnet and gloves on the floor, she fell into the chair. "I fail to understand why women cannot move about freely in Harvard Yard. We pay tuition for our education, we enroll in the same courses, we have the same expectations. It is 1892. Yet we are denied this very basic freedom *to walk in a yard*. What is the fear?"

Hoisting herself from the heavy oak chair, Elizabeth, with her massive dark brown crinoline skirt and swept-up bustle, rose, and, walking to the front of her desk, stood before Annette. The wall-mounted frosted gas lamp behind the desk created a hazy, shadowy image of the older woman.

Taking Annette's hand in hers, Elizabeth sighed, stating that she knew the fear was real and that women were frightening to many men. "Mitigating such fear," she projected, "will require time and willingness on our part to play a long political game, one based on incremental gain."

"We mustn't, just yet, hang them from the trees."

Elizabeth helped Annette, now somewhat deflated, into a spare day dress she kept in an armoire in her private office. Annette's delicate five-foot-two-inch frame, with exquisitely small waist, pale oval face with light-blue eyes, was dwarfed in Elizabeth's dress. Her thick, straight chestnut-brown hair spilled over her shoulders.

Elizabeth had learned, long ago, that having a spare dress ready was better than knowing the reason why it was needed. Although the dress swamped her, Annette was dry, and her rage was quelled for the moment.

At her desk in a classroom with eight students, Annette was in her element. Frequently tucking the excessive crinoline from the day dress that Elizabeth had provided her under her legs, Annette was once again the smartest student in the class. Her familiarity with the classics was incomparable. From 1888 to 1890, while attending the Cambridge School for Girls established by Arthur Gilman as a preparatory school for college, Annette gained exceptional fluency in Greek, with Latin her specialty. Two years later at the Harvard Annex, she was rapidly becoming a classics scholar.

While she relished the classics, today Annette pushed back unsettling thoughts about the Annex, her family, and the role she had been cast to play by both. She appreciated that her place at both the Cambridge School for Girls and the Annex was consequent to her parents' expectation that her older brother Philip Sydney, one year her senior, attend Harvard University. To assure that Philip would attend Harvard, as did their father Amos Kidder Fiske, the family moved from New York City to Cambridge, purchasing a two-story home built in 1830 with four bedrooms, a modern water closet, cobblestone backyard paths, sitting and dining rooms, and a stable. Annette's father, a well-respected newspaper reporter and columnist, wrote for *The New York Times* and *The Boston Daily Globe*. Her mother, Caroline Child, was a native to Massachusetts, viewing herself as a Boston Brahmin. The environment was charming, conducive to a peaceful and secure, financially sheltered life.

If I were male, she knew, I would be in Harvard today, not the Annex. I would be dry, having driven my bicycle across the Harvard Yard. Albeit learned in the classics, my path is unmistakable, predictable — teaching, marriage, children, and subservience. Women are valuable and easily replaceable.

Annette was the first to recite in Latin several passages from Book One of Ovid's *Metamorphoses*, a narrative poem written in 8 BC that she had come to admire because it told the story of everything while itself defying classification. She enjoyed Ovid's epic poem — considered his magnum opus — with themes of love and the inevitability of change, that both was, and was not, an epic. Her classmates, nine in all, listened carefully to her recitation, hopeful for an error they could correct. Women in college courses were rare, and competition among them fierce in classrooms, and beyond. She wondered if students believed that their success in coursework was meaningful only if accompanied by the failure of others.

Annette had read Caesar while at the Cambridge School, among other major works. New to neither Latin nor the demanding expectations of classics teachers, Annette had been thoroughly prepared by her previous education to excel at the Annex. In her study of ancient languages, Annette had learned far more than the ability to translate, acquiring appreciation for cultures, religions, and politics. In conversations with Arthur Gilman, founder of the Cambridge School, Annette found that learning war strategies and tactics was inevitable if one read Julius Caesar carefully and thoroughly. Annette ranked first at graduation from the Cambridge School.

She had every intention to do the same at the Annex.

Classwork completed for the day, Annette changed into her now-dry shattered dress and bonnet hanging in Elizabeth's private office. Elizabeth, fond of her vivacious, spunky student, queried Annette about her classes. Was she enjoying the classics? What other courses did she plan to take?

"I enjoy the classics. I never tire reading of Roman culture and life, their government, art, entertainment, and sexual attitudes and behaviors." Tying on her still-damp bonnet, Annette turned to directly face Elizabeth. "I enjoyed our conversation today. Both you and Ovid speak of change, a very titillating word. Someday, perhaps soon, I will bicycle throughout Harvard Yard. Thank you for your encouragement — *and* for your day dress!"

Elizabeth, smiling, placed a hand gently on Annette's shoulder, saying "I am here for you. I enjoy thoughtful, provocative conversations. Let us talk more frequently."

Walking alongside her broken bicycle, Annette made the short, quarter-mile journey home under a soggy, dreary, gray sky.

She felt oddly exhilarated.

Once home, Annette retreated to her bedroom. Classics homework required privacy, concentration. As she placed her book, *De Re Publica* by Cicero, on her small desk facing her southern window, Annette felt calm after the events of the day. Gathering her steel pen, slice of potato on a small dish for cleaning the pen tip, and a porcelain inkwell, Annette aligned her writing tablet, fine white paper produced by a wood pulp press, with her pen on the left side of her desk to accommodate left-handed script. While left-handedness was no longer viewed as a sign of the devil, it did create smudges on her fine, expensive paper.

As she prepared, Annette thought of Emily Dickinson, whose poetry and lifestyle she was introduced to by Elizabeth Agassiz during an Annex book club session earlier that year. Fascinated with the lady in white's evocative themes and cloistered life, Annette imagined that her window desk would please Emily, with only nature to admire and birds to enjoy. From under her burgundy leather desk writing pad, Annette pulled out a small, single paper. On it, she had meticulously written Emily's poem published in 1858, "Nobody Knows This Little Rose" — twelve lines of poetry that set the tone for Annette's work. With a soft breeze playing against her face, Annette readied herself to read, and to translate, passages from Cicero. Slipping the poem back under her writing pad, Annette transitioned from Emily to Cicero, re-engaging in the Roman world she relished. While translation took time, she knew it would be pleasurable.

Peacefulness was short.

Marguerite, Annette's younger sister, now sixteen, flew into Annette's room, circling her arms around her sister's head, covering her mouth. "You mustn't tell anyone this, Annie, but I just heard Philip tell Momma that he has a girlfriend! Her name is Abigail, and she lives here in Cambridge. He hopes to marry her after he graduates this year from Harvard." Cheeks aglow with excitement, Margie — her nickname given to her by Annette — hoisted her sister from her desk and waltzed around the bedroom, gleefully singing "The Drinking Song" from the opera *La Traviata*.

"Philip is in love! Oh, isn't that wonderful?"

"Abigail?" repeated Annette. "How *very* New England!"

Annette was unsure if this announcement was wonderful, but she loved Margie and happily waltzed around the room with her.

Annette was a middle child. With Philip her senior and Marguerite her junior, Annette secretly enjoyed the anonymity of her position within the family. Burdened by the pressure of succeeding at Harvard, Philip, a rather fragile young man, fell ill in his first year, requiring his father to take him on a three-month trip through Cuba, Mexico, and the Pacific coast to restore his health. Quiet and somber, Philip disliked his sisters — Marguerite for her frivolity and Annette for her scholarship.

His sisters returned his dismissal.

Rarely were the three seen together. The family dined together only at holidays and major family dinners, a situation that satisfied all.

Annette's mother Caroline, however, felt the guilt of a discordant family. While unable to legitimately trace her family lineage to the Massachusetts Bay Colony, she represented herself as a Boston Brahmin. As a child, Caroline was a model of etiquette, engaging with her two brothers in all family gatherings, placing family interests above all else. Francis James, twelve years her senior, was known as Stubby, so nicknamed for his short stature by his peers at Harvard, where he became professor of rhetoric and oratory. While she adored her older, academic brother, Caroline felt painfully awkward in the presence of his stately wife, Elizabeth Ellen Sedgwick, for reasons she did not fully understand. Caroline did not endorse her sister-in-law's activities, wondering why her eminent brother tolerated her questionable ventures with unsavory people. At family gatherings, Caroline would go to great lengths to avoid sitting next to Elizabeth at the dinner table. William, Caroline's eldest sibling, a leather merchant operating a successful business in Boston, was generally unwilling to participate in family gatherings, citing conflicts with work.

Proud of her place in Boston elite society as wife and homemaker, Caroline found it difficult to imprint her values on her daughters. Neither Annette nor Marguerite voiced interest in homemaking. Both demanded education, but their paths were deviant to her — one desirous of becoming an opera singer and the other a classics scholar. Neither flirted with boys nor spoke of first loves. Neither enjoyed cooking or baking, seeing these kitchen activities only as necessary chores best conducted by others. As a young girl, Annette never played with her mother's jewelry nor dressed in her fancy gowns. And, although Annette was grooming herself as a scholar, she did so with a future career goal in mind rather than to simply be an educated mother for her children.

Caroline feared the influence of the newly founded General Federation of Women's Clubs on Annette — groups of outspoken women advocating women's suffrage, prohibition, child labor laws, and more. Worse, the National American Woman Suffrage Association claimed that men and women were equal members of society. These views appalled Caroline. Clearly, she thought, men and women were not equals — how could they be? They had different functions in polite society, one securing income and the other maintaining homes. Caroline worried that such organizations threatened the very institution of marriage.

When she thought of Philip, however, Caroline sighed with relief. Philip would soon graduate with his Harvard degree, obtain a position in business or journalism, and start a family. She was proud of Philip. He had chosen the proper path. And now, he spoke of Abigail, or Abbie as he called her, as the love of his life.

To solidify Philip's path, Caroline planned an afternoon tea to introduce Abbie to her daughters and her own siblings and their families. Annette and Marguerite were pressed into service, Marguerite to entertain guests with songs from operettas, Annette to help the kitchen maids prepare the baking.

To Annette's delight, if not her mother's, her Aunt Elizabeth had promised to attend the little celebration. Elizabeth oftentimes avoided family events, claiming her community work took precedence. Although unsure of what community work meant, Annette knew to avoid this topic at tea, having been coached by her mother that her aunt's services oftentimes dealt with unpleasant subjects and people from a different class.

Elizabeth intrigued Annette.

Replacing Cicero with baking, Annette quietly undertook her designated tasks. As her taste-tester, Annette's father, Amos, congratulated her on delicious cookies and muffins. A thin man with thick gray hair, a craggy face, and rimless glasses teetering unsteadily on the bridge of his nose, Amos was generally seen with a steel pen in his right hand and a small notecard in his left hand. "Jot down your meaningful thoughts as you have them," he once told Annette. "You may not remember them later." Words were his stock in trade, indeed his livelihood. Orphaned and penniless at sixteen, his work at a cotton mill in his birth state of New Hampshire earned him enough income to enroll in Appleton Academy, a private school chartered in 1789. A self-made journalist and lawyer, Amos first earned his Harvard degree and subsequently, his law credential, becoming a journalist who wrote his way to prestigious posts at both *The Globe* and *The Times*.

"Annie, you are a magnificent baker! Your husband will be a very happy man!"

Annette frowned, avoiding his wistful gaze.

"Father, baking is one thing, marriage another." They left the kitchen, strolling slowly to the gazebo in their graveled backyard pungent with the aroma of rose bushes meticulously planted by her mother. There they sat, uneasily looking at each other.

"Your mother has begun to explore suitors for you. When you graduate in two years, we assume that you will marry, have children and a home of your own. Is this not what you want?"

Amos was not surprised at his daughter's quiet reticence, having never sensed in her the desire for homemaking, nor family life. He feared that such a life would bore her, increasingly so as she advanced her education. Yet, what did she want? Amos knew never to assume, but deviating from this particular assumption would be radically disruptive to his wife.

"I am unsure of what I want my life to be; it is too soon to know. I am unsure of who I am yet," Annette said to a nearby rosebush.

They returned to the house, which was beginning to fill with guests. A contrast to Philip, Abigail was lovely, with a plumpness and animated, large spirit that enlivened her brother. Far from shy, she soon orchestrated the dinner conversation, directing roles for all to play at the table. Caroline's cheeks flushed with delight. Finally, here was a daughter bred for marriage and family.

Once tea had been enjoyed and the table cleared, guests entered the sitting parlor, with Marguerite commanding attention with her soprano performance of Verdi's *Sempre Libera.* As directed by Caroline, Annette served tea in delicate, bone-colored China cups, each with different intricate, translucent floral patterns. Blueberry scones and raisin biscuits were set on eggshell Georgian bread plates.

Marguerite planned to become a special, non-degree student at the Harvard Annex in a few months. She dreamed of fluency in Italian and Spanish, the so-called modern languages she deemed beautiful, ideal for operas and travel abroad. Mesmerizing the room, Marguerite had fully captured her audience, all spellbound by her robust voice and piano magic. Music lessons, thought Caroline, had paid off for Marguerite. A beauty already at sixteen, Marguerite was taller than her sister, with a fuller figure and long, curly auburn hair framing her face, highlighting deep hazel eyes. Frequently mistaken as Spanish, Marguerite relished the zarzuela, Spain's national style of opera. Surely, Caroline forecast, Marguerite's musical skills, complemented by her beauty, would someday attract an eligible suitor.

Annette joined her Uncle Stubby and Aunt Elizabeth, who had ventured to a small library adjoining the sitting parlor once Marguerite completed her first solo set. "Home at last!" Stubby exclaimed, smiling at his smart, young niece. Stubby noted that his English and Scottish ballads held a prominent position in the bookcase close to the fireplace. "Annette, I was fortunate that Charlie Eliot named me Harvard's first Professor of English. He gave me a special gift—time! I conducted my research for the ballads without ever reading students' papers. Can you imagine?" His gleeful statement was rhetorical, yet Stubby noted a sulky expression on Annette's face in return. Known within the family for his often-unpredictable statements, Stubby angled to engage his niece in a conversation.

"Do you see yourself teaching when you graduate, Annette? If not teaching, then what?"

Saying that she no more wished to read students' papers than he did, Annette fell silent.

"You will surely marry, correct?" Stubby was grasping, unsure of his next words and fearful to offend his prickly niece.

"Marriage, Uncle, is not an occupation."

Excusing herself, Annette ventured to the door of the library. Before she could leave, her Aunt Elizabeth had tapped her shoulder, asking her to take the fresh air for a few minutes.

Annette and Elizabeth left together, Annette irascible and Elizabeth distraught as she rummaged in her dress pocket for a cigarette. Stubby remained in the library, content and comfortable in a large easy chair with soft side arms, smiling contentedly as he thumbed through his own work, *The English and Scottish Popular Ballads*.

"Smoke?" Elizabeth lit a Vanity Fair cigarette, complete with mouthpiece, and handed it to Annette. Inhaling deeply, Annette's face reddened, immediately followed by strenuous gasping. Expressing thanks to her aunt, she fingered the cigarette in her hand, seeming unwilling to return it.

"Keep it. You are now inaugurated into the suffrage movement!" Elizabeth laughed, explaining that ladies' cigarettes had become an infamous symbol of the suffrage movement. "Yes, marriage is not an occupation. You are correct." Commenting that she advocated for women's right to vote, Elizabeth said she smoked far more than she should, risking respiratory illness in favor of equal rights.

Chuckling, Annette watched as her sixty-eight-year-old her aunt tucked her cigarettes down deeply into her dress pocket.

"Annette, call me Ellen. My middle name is actually Ellery, but I prefer Ellen. Elizabeth is so very British, so royal. Like you, I value my occupation, and my independence. I am a suffragist. I fight for my cause, as did my grandfather, Theodore Sedgwick. He was a major in the Continental Army during the American Revolution, later becoming a U. S. senator and then, a U. S. representative from Massachusetts. Theodore pleaded a slave's suit for freedom from her owners, claiming that the 1780 Massachusetts constitution held that all men are born equal and free. He won the case. More than a century later, do you think my grandfather would think women equal and free in our society?"

Not expecting a response, Ellen shifted tone, inviting Annette to join her the next day at a regional meeting of the General Federation of Women's Clubs. The meeting was to be held in the Boston home of the local chapter president, Claire Williams, secretary for her husband's law firm. Since the next day was Saturday, Annette, stifling overt enthusiasm, said she was pleased to join her.

"It's settled then," stated Ellen. "I'll have you picked up at noon. Wear comfortable clothing."

"Should I bring anything?" Annette asked.

With a twinkle in her eyes, Ellen replied: "Yes, backbone."

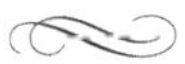

Claire's Victorian brownstone home on Beacon Street was built in 1817, in the Back Bay neighborhood of Boston, adjacent to Cambridge. With a red brick exterior, brown shuttered windows, and arched front with heavy oak double doors, the structure was impressive. The gardens were equally so, with red and orange chrysanthemums adorning each step of the front porch and ornamental flowering purple kale and cream-colored cabbage bordering the house's base.

Annette and Ellen's driver pulled on the reigns, bringing the two horses to a halt immediately at the double doors. Both side doors of the dark-blue, four-wheeled brougham carriage opened, the driver assisting Ellen to alight elegantly. Annette cautiously stepped from the carriage, struggling to appear composed and confident. Scanning the large, worn semi-circular cobblestone driveway, she counted twelve similar carriages, with drivers gathered in a nearby gazebo, enjoying their chewing tobacco, pipes, and cigars.

The last carriage entering the driveway was a one-horse hansom cab with a single passenger, Frances Willard. Annette recognized her from pictures published in the *Women's Journal and Suffrage News*, a periodical founded in 1870 by Lucy Stone, a suffragist, in Boston. Annette's classmates routinely distributed the weekly newspaper within the Annex, with the endorsement of Elizabeth Agassiz. Such a prominent figure, Annette mused, wondering now about the relationships between and among Ellen, Elizabeth Agassiz, and Frances Willard.

What was the purpose of the meeting at Claire's home?

"Frances," Claire said as she held her guest's hand to help her step down from the cab, "thank you so very much for joining us today. Our agenda is full, so I'll escort you now to our main sitting parlor."

Frances smiled warmly, waving to other guests as she and Claire approached the entranceway. At fifty-three, Frances was a formidable presence, despite her small stature, long oval face, gracious smile, and warm slate-blue eyes. Perhaps, thought Annette, Frances's middle-parted hair pulled tightly in an upward sweeping bun, her rimless eyeglasses held intact by a neck chain, and her vertical posture were intentionally designed to culminate in a serious, almost stern, appearance. Only vaguely aware of Willard's social activism, Annette thought it wise to remain silent during any subsequent discussions, fearful of the disdain that might accompany her ignorance of the current women's movement.

As Claire's sixteen guests gathered in the main parlor, servants began offering light tea sandwiches of ham and mustard, cucumber, and egg and watercress, followed by petite lemon cream custard biscuits. Guests appreciated the light fare, gathering in small groups of two or three, enjoying each other's company in private conversations prior to the start of the meeting. Annette was struck by the camaraderie of the women at this high tea, all of whom were animated, in fact, quite lively.

As a group, they exuded confidence, speaking in voices louder than she had ever heard women speak before. Two older guests sat together in a red velvet chesterfield chaise lounge sofa, holding hands, engaged in a private conversation. Perhaps, Annette wondered, were these women in a Boston marriage, or, as her mother would have described them, unmarried spinsters? Annette had learned of lesbianism at the Cambridge School through her reading of Greek poetry. The fluid sexuality of Greeks was inextricably interlaced with the cosmos, the earth, and Hades. Lesbianism in the ancient world was also examined at the Annex, with Annette encountering several classmates inviting engagements, which she declined.

The openness of the two women sitting closely in the chaise lounge in Claire's home intrigued Annette. Immersed in the prudishness of the Back Bay, Annette was perhaps even more surprised by the acceptance of women in love by the other guests. Claire's home was a safe place, something apart from the censorious legal system and chilly society beyond her great doors.

The agenda for the regional General Federation of Women's Clubs was disguised as short, listing only two action items, concluding with a summary update of future directions. "First, let me introduce our main speaker, Miss Frances Willard, president of the Women's Christian Temperance Union, a position she has held since 1879. She will address the relationships among suffrage, social housekeeping, prohibition, birth control, and public health. Thank you, Frances, for traveling to be with us today." Claire applauded, with all present joining in. The two guests in the chaise lounge chair stood and cheered. Frances stood and nodded, then returned quietly to her seat, smiling at the women in the lounge chair.

Claire provided background regarding the first action item, support for Mary Philbrook, a young New Jersey woman who intended to take the bar examination to become a lawyer. Since the New Jersey Court had determined that a woman did not have the right to practice as an attorney, Mary was not allowed to sit for the bar examination. "Mary," Claire stated, "needs our club's support." Turning to Lelia Robinson and Anna Christy Fall, invited guests, Claire asked them to review their experiences in becoming lawyers in Massachusetts.

Robinson, the first female admitted to the bar in Massachusetts, spoke first, recalling that she had graduated from Boston University School of Law in 1881, the only woman in a class of 150. Leading a campaign to enable women to take the bar exam and practice law in Massachusetts, Robinson noted that she had successfully argued that men *and women* were citizens under the state's bar statute, and thus, entitled to take the legal exam. Robinson succeeded in her argument, cleverly avoiding conflation of the bar exam with women's right to suffrage, a topic anathema to politicians.

Similarly, Anna Fall recalled that she had graduated magna cum laude in 1891 from Boston University School of Law and, in that same year, became the first woman to try, and win, a jury case in Massachusetts. She noted that she was the first female lawyer to argue a case before the state's supreme court. She stressed the need for women nationally to support Mary Philbrook in her plea to sit for the bar examination in New Jersey, a state with, as she characterized them, "draconian practices relative to admitting women to legal practice."

Claire then raised the question: "What, specifically, do you want from our club?"

"Support," responded Robinson. "An official letter of support from your club to the New Jersey legislature, addressing the urgency to pass a bill enabling women to take the bar examination."

Claire, seeking a vote to send a letter of support as requested, was not surprised with the unanimous endorsement of the motion. Recognizing that one letter would not be enough to even be noticed, Claire indicated that she would inform all clubs in Massachusetts to write similar letters, using their club's letter as a model.

"It is truly time to take action!" Claire knew that legislatures needed to be inundated, perhaps even overwhelmed, with information if an item was to be noticed. Power, she knew, was driven by action.

Annette, attentive to the previous motion, was now lightheaded, a bit off-balance in terms of the foreign tone and context of the women's world she had now entered. While the request for a letter of support was rational to her, the female ambiance of the club was disquieting, unfamiliar. What is expected of club members? As a club member, would I be required to formulate my individual opinion on any specific matter and then defend that opinion publicly? Unsure, Annette looked at her aunt's profile, seeking understanding in her facial expression. Yes, she reasoned, club members examine information, take stands on important matters, and then act. Words without action are useless. As to the openness of the lesbian women in the club, Annette assumed a Greek indifference to sexuality, holding the belief that sexuality and sexual behaviors were private matters.

After the motion was endorsed, a brief break followed, with Ellen and Annette sitting in wide rocking chairs on the large porch. Ellen enjoyed her cigarette, lifting her face to the sky to feel the light warm breeze. Annette, squelching a cough, took a long drag on her cigarette, eager to appear a seasoned smoker.

"Annette," Ellen said softly, in a conspiratorial tone, "we—women—must contribute to society. Listen carefully to Frances Willard, and ask questions if you wish, given that your own future is being determined now, but not by you, by your mother." Ellen offered that she and Stubby, Annette's uncle, were quite different, but tolerant of each other's need to remain independent and to contribute separately to society. "If you are to be a wife, then look for a partner rather than a husband. Read Harriet Beecher Stowe, who wrote that a married woman can make no contract and hold no property—in common law, a married woman is nothing at all. So, certainly, you will teach the classics upon graduation."

"Or," Ellen added, "you may explore the world you see here today, and think of your place in it."

Perhaps for the first time, Annette recognized just how dangerous Ellen appeared to her mother. Harboring heretical views of women, inciting women to action, and promoting a wife's life as independent from her husband's, Ellen was following in her grandfather Theodore Sedgwick's steps. Like him, Ellen was a revolutionary. He had fought for his country's independence, and she, for women's independence. Even her appearance, Annette realized, screamed of non-conformity. With wiry grayish-white hair loosely held by a ribbon in a long ponytail that she curled over her left shoulder, and wearing a shortened pale-blue day dress over a pair of lacy, billowy dark-blue pants, Ellen was easily labeled a bloomer, an advocate of dress reform for women.

Bloomers and cigarettes.

"Ellen," asked Annette, "where do you purchase your bloomers?"

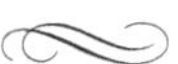

Frances Willard, set of small note cards in her left hand, walked noiselessly within Claire Williams' large sitting parlor, where club members were seated, captivated by her expressive face. Angry for not bringing blank note cards to the meeting, Annette focused her attention and excellent memory fastidiously on Frances's language. I will write key points in my tablet once home, she thought.

"Legalized traffic in strong drink devastates families."

"Intoxicated men commit violent acts against women, including rape." Without the right to vote, Frances claimed, women remained powerless, their homes unprotected, their health assailed, their days defined by household servitude. She spoke of home protection, a phrase endorsed by clubs nationally to couple women's suffrage to crimes committed by drunken men. Through the vote, there would be consequences for brutal crimes against women.

"The right to vote," Frances said, "assures equality between men and women. Until we vote, women will remain the incumbrance and toy of men."

Frowning, Ellen shifted restlessly in her chair. "Frances," she asked, "is not the movement more encompassing than the thread of home protection? Societal protection, higher education for women, employment opportunities, and birth control options—are these factors included in the mantra *home protection*?"

As if dealing with an overly enthusiastic child, Frances gently placed her hand on Ellen's shoulder. "Ellen, we aim for equal rights under the law. All that you mention must be included. We must, however, be strategic. Not all women, as you know, desire to vote. Encouraging such to demand birth control would be a foolhardy use of time at present. Incremental wins, that is how politics works well. We can legislate birth control if we can vote."

"You must understand that the average woman lives to forty-eight years of age and gives birth to between seven and eight children, often in under ten years. While managing pregnancy, birth, and childcare, she is also maintaining a household, cooking, cleaning, mending, shopping, and more." Allowing her glasses to slip off her face and dangle around her neck on her eyeglass retainer, she added, in a slow voice, that "a mother may also be warding off sexual advances from a drunken husband." Such a woman, commonly uneducated, owning no property, having no income, had no rights under the law.

"Annette, you seem quizzical." Frances smiled at Annette, adding that "change depends on actions of young women such as yourself."

Perturbed at being singled out, Annette stood up, never one to be challenged or second guessed.

"Quizzical, no, but puzzled. I need your help to better understand the priorities you are describing." Annette continued, seeking clarity on women's voting priorities. Which is more critical, birth control or prohibition of alcohol? Can laws be passed concurrently? Are there currently protections against multiple, unwanted pregnancies? Eager for understanding, Annette stimulated discussion on solutions to protect women from violent, perhaps drunken husbands. Prohibition of alcohol, birth control, both?

Spent by her own animation, Annette took her seat, cheeks aglow. Ellen smiled broadly at Frances, proud of her niece.

"Annette, you are correct. Prohibition of alcohol and birth control are needed at the same time. *Now!*" Frances, surprised yet intrigued by Annette's straightforward language, continued, stating that birth control was crucial if women were to contribute to society beyond the home.

She scanned the room, assessing her listeners' reactions. Sensing more agreement than trepidation, Frances continued. "Pregnancy is exhausting, and multiple pregnancies drain a woman. And, while homemade abortion remedies continue surreptitiously, recall that abortion is not birth control. Our Comstock Act remains in force, and physicians are unable to mail either birth control information or devices to patients. We need to advocate for the right to vote and for effective birth control. Without these, women will continue as toys in the hands of men."

Needing more information, Lelia Robinson, forever the lawyer, asked if home protection equated with social housekeeping, the latter the mantra of the General Federation of Women's Clubs. Novice to this language, Annette whispered to Ellen, "Why are these phrases viewed as critical?"

"Phrases become rallying cries," said Ellen, "truisms worthy of battle." She explained that everything Frances addressed — from voting to birth control, to owning property, to education — would be subsumed in a simple chant.

"Annette, did not Caesar have a rallying cry? It was he who galvanized his soldiers to war with 'Cry *havoc*' and 'Let slip the dogs of war!'"

While Annette understood that it was Marc Antony who chanted these phrases in Shakespeare's play, she did not correct her aunt.

Yes, she thought, recoiling with some embarrassment for her aunt, I understand the havoc's cry. Earlier, Frances had said simply "Do everything" to achieve women's causes as promoted by the Women's Christian Temperance Union. She advocated war. This, Annette understood, was Frances's desire to let the dogs slip on the social order, to ultimately free women.

For Annette, however, the variables seemed more complex than prohibition and birth control. Frances was not telling the complete story. Recently, her Annex book club had reviewed Charles Dickens' 1853 book *Bleak House*, with one classmate, Sadie, comparing the damage emanating from wealth—the "illth," as coined by John Ruskin—to the poverty and degradation of poor farming plebeians and slaves in ancient Rome. Sadie had postulated that poverty, crowding, malnutrition, disease, addiction, and mud (in actuality, feces) permeating the streets of London may have also deeply pervaded the lives of the lower classes in Rome. While not defining herself as a social activist, Sadie had been vibrant and animated in her translation of several passages from Cicero's work. How did poverty, crowding, and disease feature in Frances's story, Annette wondered?

While not an avid reader of health news, Annette was obliquely aware of Lemuel Shattuck's 1850 report on the sanitary condition of Massachusetts, given her father's bent toward investigative journalism and articles on infection and sanitary science. What was glaringly omitted in Frances's narrative was disease.

Claire spoke, breaking Annette's reverie.

"What action, Frances, do you propose we take at this time?"

Returning to Lelia Robinson's question, Frances equated home protection with social housekeeping, given that both phrases implied similar goals. To "do everything" required social reform, with women's suffrage paramount.

"What to do next?" Frances posed rhetorically.

"Information is power. Be informed. Stay informed. Spread information on suffrage. Read the *Woman's Journal*. Participate in rallies, attend programs on voting, birth control, prohibition. Never stop advocating for, and working toward, the right to vote."

Without hesitation, Annette raised her hand.

"What of diseases spread by sexual intimacy? What of the connections among birth control, infections spread through sexual intimacy, pregnancy, and women's health? What other actions can be taken *now* to prevent pregnancy as well as disease spread by intimacy?"

Frances paused, listening intensely to Annette's passionate voice, taken with the girl's courage in addressing such subjects.

"Condoms. We can advocate for aggressive production and distribution of condoms. This will also take much education, as men may not want to use condoms." Frances was straightforward, almost casual. "It will also require women to say *no* to unprotected sex. Again, as with men and condom use, we will need to educate women in this regard. Men and women must change behaviors, with women championing this change. We must be courageous, with or without the right to vote. Protected sex must become our norm."

In summary, Claire detailed two actions to be taken. First, support of women's suffrage and second, advocacy for use of male condoms.

Although unsatisfied with this summary, bland as it was, Annette was silent. I am a guest, she thought. Perhaps I have already said enough. Glancing at Ellen, deep in conversation with both Claire and Frances, she imagined that she might not be invited back. On the journey home, Ellen sought Annette's thoughts on the meeting.

"I am glad to have been there," Annette said enthusiastically.

She expressed some uncertainty about next steps to achieve the Do Everything agenda but noted that the Annex book club was a vehicle to introduce new, provocative ideas. Since the club would meet next week, Annette agreed to select a book consistent with the Do Everything agenda, even if only in a tangential way. Advocates, she knew, would be best approached delicately, with sensibilities respected.

Wanting closure on the day, Annette shut her eyes, hoping Ellen would accept silence. "I hope you'll join me again for the next Club meeting," Ellen said as she placed her hand on Annette's shoulder. "You contributed much today. You took risks. I am proud of you!"

Annette smiled at Ellen, hoping to nap uninterrupted.

"I would be pleased to attend the next Women's Club meeting with you, Annette."

Elizabeth Agassiz smiled at her protégé, recalling that she was a founding member of the General Federation of Women's Clubs, begun in 1890.

"Organization is power, Annette. You will do well to remember that." The older woman rose from her large Victorian-style walnut armchair and selected a book from the floor-to-ceiling bookcase behind her desk. Her heavy silk brocade taffeta dress swept the floor — making a faint *swish* sound — as she turned to the bookcase. Always prepared for company, Elizabeth wore brocade, muslin, or linen dresses with accompanying shawls and decorative headbands daily. She loved clothes, and gradually wore fancier dresses after her husband's death in 1873, the year of Annette's birth.

Elizabeth rarely spoke of Louis Agassiz, who she had married in 1850 shortly after the death of his first wife. A renowned Harvard professor of zoology and geology, Louis was, according to Elizabeth, a complex man — productive, driven, and demanding. Throughout their marriage, Elizabeth assisted him in his academic pursuits, particularly preparing publications. As his views of polygenism evolved, Elizabeth came to believe him cruel. Exposed to his indifferent, careless treatment of people of different races, most evidenced by daguerreotypes of Renty Taylor, a slave, Elizabeth began to mark her independent life in the final years of their marriage.

The older woman noticed that Annette was watching her carefully. Elizabeth wondered if Annette thought she was about to select a book of her husband's.

"In his later career, my husband considered Whites the superior race. Since my life followed his, that period was frightening and lonely. I have lived only after his death."

"Dress as you will, Annette," Elizabeth advised, smoothing out a wrinkle in her large, flouncy skirt. In how many ways had Louis constrained her life?

"And accomplish *your* goals." Sensing that Elizabeth seemed poised to say more, Annette was silent.

Elizabeth placed a legal-sized, leather-bound journal, tied with leather lacing, into Annette's hands. The journal was Elizabeth's private diary, housing original documents and correspondence related to her role in the 1879 establishment of the Society for the Private Collegiate Instruction of Women and her directorship of the Harvard Annex. Letters to and from Harvard president

Charles W. Eliot and other Society and Annex administrators were meticulously catalogued. Pictures and other memorabilia were securely tucked in a mailing envelope in the back pouch of the journal.

"I am honored to hold your journal." Honored, but uncertain as to why she was given it, Annette said that she would read the documents if Elizabeth would allow her to take it home for private reading.

"You can certainly read it and return it to me when you are finished. You may also wish it to serve as a focus point for a future Annex book club discussion. Women need to hear the story of women. Women must find their voices, determine who they are, what they wish to contribute. At a local level, the book club can accomplish what the Women's Clubs do at a larger, societal level. I can join you at your next book club meeting, if your peers wish to invite me. And, since I am a member of the Women's Club managed by Claire Williams, I can also join you at their next meeting. Will your Aunt Elizabeth attend also?"

Elizabeth had returned to her armchair, almost breathless, as if frightened. Will my legacy be honored? She questioned herself, unsure of her own motives. She did, however, know that her journal contained documents of historical significance to women, a thought giving her solace. Elizabeth considered Annette a reliable, trustworthy heir to all the journal represented.

Annette stated that she was eager to call the next book club meeting, to be determined on Elizabeth's availability. Still feeling the loss of her journal, Elizabeth regained her composure, apprising Annette of her calendar. "My journal, Annette," remarked Elizabeth, "must be understood simply as a symbol of women's independence. Such independence is powerful, and often best expressed through organizations. That is what I wish you and your peers to recognize through your discussions of my journal." Elizabeth was spent. Feeling as if she had manumitted her legacy, Elizabeth left her office with Annette, journal safely packed in the younger woman's bookbag.

Once home, Annette contacted Ellen, informing her in excited tones that President Agassiz would join them at Claire's next club meeting.

Eager to open Elizabeth's leather journal, Annette sat at her window desk, recalling the first verse of yet another Emily Dickinson poem, published just one year earlier:

That perches in the soul,
And sings the tune without the words,
And never stops at all, . . .

As Annette placed Elizabeth's bound journal safely on her desk by the window, Caroline, her mother, created a schedule for Annette's courtship. She was a meticulous planner, every detail considered, including Annette's hair jewelry to be worn at a dinner party next week. What, indeed, would be a successful outcome? Caroline contemplated. A courtship begun, with plans for marriage in the near future, was the goal. While oftentimes labeled a dreamer, Caroline knew her daughter, and realized that the road to its end might be bumpy and take a bit longer than she wished. She found solace, however, in her thoughts of Marguerite, Annette's younger, vivacious sibling. Margie, as her siblings called her, already had suitors at sixteen years of age, a comforting thought for a mother whose goal was for her daughters to marry well. Caroline's preparations for Annette's courtship would not have been wasted if the intended fiancé, Alistair Campbell, married *either* Annette *or* Marguerite.

Alistair Campbell, twenty-two, a recent Harvard graduate focusing on finance, planned a life in banking, his goal to be a bank executive. Matthew Campbell, Alistair's father, was a Scottish immigrant to Boston in 1866. Known as a mathematical genius, Matthew, an engineering graduate of the University of Edinburgh, was an experienced textile mill owner and operator. At a young age, he accrued wealth and a reputation as a successful entrepreneur. As his business acumen grew, Matthew had quietly followed events in the US Civil War, anticipating that his sustained future success would occur in America. When the war ended, he and his bride, Kirstine, traveled to New York, ultimately settling in Boston. Matthew became as famous in Boston as he was in Scotland.

As his wealth grew, so did his interests, with burgeoning enjoyment of fine arts, particularly, paintings and drawings. Alistair's birth in 1870 provided Matthew the pivot needed to turn full-time to fine arts, with a recruit hired to provide daily management of his textile business while he still retained control. When the Massachusetts legislature passed an act that incorporated the Trustees of the Museum of Fine Arts in 1870, Matthew avidly followed the construction of the massive red brick and terracotta Gothic Revival-style building located in Copley Square.

Completed in 1876, the Museum of Fine Arts required a director.

Matthew applied and was interviewed by the twelve trustees. Always fascinated by things that were not quite like all others, Charles W. Eliot, president of Harvard University and a trustee of the museum, was intrigued with Campbell. Certainly, Eliot enjoyed the Scottish accent, reminiscent of his previous travels to Great Britain. He was most impressed with Matthew's combination of skills—management of a practical business, facility with math and finance, aptitude for scientific language, and ability to strategically plan. Here, thought Eliot, was the type of trained professional required for a reimagined America, a country groomed for world leadership through progressive education. If Matthew were our director, then the museum's future is assured, thought Eliot. Perhaps an invitation to join Harvard's Board of Overseers would augment an employment offer, an attractive compliment to woo Matthew to the museum.

Matthew needed little wooing. He had been thrilled to join the museum as director, and equally taken with an appointment to Harvard's Board of Overseers.

While Matthew and Kirstine planned for Alistair to be educated at Harvard, they first enrolled him in Boston Latin School, the oldest school in America, established in Boston in 1635. Like his father, Alistair did exceptionally well in school and completed his AB degree at Harvard with highest honors in 1890.

Alistair enjoyed finance, managing the books as Matthew termed it. Earning wealth, then banking it. These were themes guiding his work ethic. Indeed, he planned for a future in which his excess wealth would be disbursed in support of worthy causes. Both he and his father were deeply influenced by the essay "Wealth," a philosophy of philanthropy published in 1889 by Andrew Carnegie, the Scottish steel magnate, in the *North American Review*. While Carnegie generously supported libraries, the arts, museums, and other enterprises with his large resources, Matthew and Alistair Campbell intended to emulate his generosity on a smaller but very meaningful scale.

Matthew and Alistair planned to announce their offer of an endowed professorship of arts at Harvard University by the late

1890s. "Textiles," Matthew once said slyly to Charles Eliot, "are a very lucrative commodity."

The loyal friendship between Matthew and Charles, dating almost twenty years, enwrapped Alistair upon his graduation. Charles worked closely with the Campbells as the trio defined the structure of the endowment. Now, as Alistair launched his finance career as a young bank manager in Boston, both Matthew and Charles anticipated that he would marry and begin a family — become entrenched in the Back Bay community.

Caroline agreed with Ellen and Stubby that the dinner party to introduce Annette to Alistair would take place at Elizabeth Agassiz's home on Quincy Street, at the invitation of the Annex's president. Elizabeth's home was larger, able to accommodate at least twelve people at the dining table. For her part, Elizabeth wanted control, particularly given Caroline's sometimes erratic, flighty conversations.

Unknown to Caroline, the agenda for her planned dinner party had grown. No longer simply an opportunity to spark a courtship, the party was now a vehicle supporting a plethora of opportunities.

Ellen, Elizabeth, and Annette hoped to discuss the Women's Club plan for social activism.

Elizabeth intended to secure Charles's agreement with her goals for the Harvard Annex.

Stubby and Charles planned to introduce physician Alfred Worcester and his health agenda for the city.

And Charles, Matthew, and Alistair planned to design the skeleton structure of an endowed professorship in the arts at Harvard.

As guests arrived, Elizabeth escorted them into her spacious parlor room, brimming with comfortable armchairs, stuffed sofas, a few small end tables, grand fireplace, a piano, and a large circular center table with red roses in an ornate crystal vase. Lit by oil lamp wall sconces and infused with the sweet aroma of roses, the parlor was warm and inviting. Elizabeth's commanding voice and bustling presence was welcoming, as she deftly introduced guests new to her circle.

Annette smiled as she caught Elizabeth's gaze, pleased that her mentor had orchestrated this occasion. In a light-lavender silk gown with three-quarter sleeves and small rhinestones in the collar, Annette felt confident, almost comfortable. While not driven by the fashions of the day, Annette did appreciate gowns that accentuated her small waist, fragile arms, and flawless skin. Her light-brown hair was swept up into a neat chignon held in place loosely with a purple coral comb, with soft curls escaping around her temples. "I look," she thought, "rather Greek." Scanning the parlor quickly, she noticed only two people unfamiliar to her. Both men, one younger, perhaps in his twenties, and the other older, mid-thirties. Neither was accompanied by a female companion.

Clearly, thought Annette, the younger man may be Alistair Campbell, my intended fiancé. With average height, a lean body type, and an affable, comfortable demeanor, he easily commandeered attention in the room. Annette was drawn to his face. Lean with hazel-colored eyes, thick strawberry-blonde hair and light beard, Alistair exuded a friendly warmth that drew people to him. He was conversing with the older, taller gentleman when Annette approached.

"Hello." Annette extended her hand to Alistair, which he grasped, shaking warmly. "I am Annette," she said, without hesitation. "If you are Alistair Campbell, then I am the woman you have been brought here tonight to meet."

Seemingly caught a bit off guard, Alistair recovered, affirming that he was indeed her intended suitor. "I would like you to meet a colleague of mine, an earlier graduate of Harvard's medical school, Alfred Worcester. He is a practicing family physician in Waltham, a neighboring city about ten miles from here." Winking at Annette, Alistair added that "Alfred will explain his adventures in hospital care and nurses' training over dinner tonight." Alfred took Annette's hand in his and gently shook it, nodding his head.

Here, thought Annette, is something very different. She had connected quickly, warmly, and easily with Alistair. And she noticed the attention Alistair paid to Alfred, with perhaps too-long glances.

Alfred was quieter, more aloof, a foreigner displaced in Elizabeth's parlor. Still a member of Harvard's alumni network, but in a field so different as to make him unusual. Alistair and Alfred were both out of the ordinary, but for contrasting reasons. Alfred's light slate-blue eyes were piercing, his middle-parted hair curled by his ears and at his neck, his oval face smooth without mustache or beard. Annette did not notice the wedding ring on his left hand.

As guests began to take their seats at the dinner table, Elizabeth announced the final guest. Charles Eliot, president of Harvard, was ushered into the dining hall, hat and greatcoat taken by a housemaid. By virtue of his status, Charles sat at one end of the table, with Elizabeth at the opposite end. Both presidents, one of Harvard and the other of Harvard Annex. Class status was a prominent factor in the social order in Back Bay culture. Caroline sat next to Elizabeth, with Amos, her husband, at her side. Annette sat next to Alistair, whose father, Matthew, sat opposite them with Ellen, Stubby, and Alfred.

The delightful aromas infusing the dining room were intoxicating to the guests, momentarily caught off guard by the hostess's dinner. Lit only by the two majestic table candelabras, the room was warm and inviting. As the guests took their assigned seats, two kitchen maids served winter vegetable soup in classic Royal Albert Wedgwood China, robust with carrots, turnips, onions, potatoes, celery, and a rich variety of herbs, most notably parsley and sage. As one kitchen maid ladled steamy winter vegetable soup into delicate bowls, a second maid poured pinot noir into Waterford wine glasses. The aroma of sweet herbal winter soup filled the room. The setting was idyllic for polite discussion, with a large table centerpiece of fresh-cut roses anchored on either side by five-candle ornately decorated silver candelabras, long tapers brightening the table.

As if dictated by a stage manager, Charles and Elizabeth began act one over soup. Tall, even in his chair, Charles was regal, with a long, straight nose, steel-framed spectacles, a violet-colored birthmark on his right cheek partially obscured by a muttonchop beard, and a heavily starched collar. Charles was thirty-five when installed as president of Harvard University in 1869. Deeply influenced by events of the Civil War, Charles proposed higher education as indispensable preparation for America's role as world leader. By 1892, he had moved the Harvard Corporation rapidly to his goal of all fields of study at their best.

Tonight, Charles felt grateful to Elizabeth. She had planned for dinner to be held on Saturday, not Sunday. At his request, however, Elizabeth shifted the event to Sunday. Her friend Charlie, as Elizabeth referred to him privately, abhorred Sundays, a day his family attended two services in King's Chapel on Tremont Street in Boston during his youth. With playing games forbidden on Sundays, and only *good* books approved, Charles had felt trapped, longing for nighttime and a chance to read the latest Waverley novel. Despite poor eyesight, Charles survived Sundays with his friends Walter Scott and Charles Dickens. From childhood on, Sundays bored Charles. The dinner party would provide a welcome night out.

Charles intended to enjoy the evening.

"Thank you, Elizabeth, for choreographing our dinner." Nodding to Elizabeth, Charles signaled for her to officiate, which she did with great aplomb.

Alert to Caroline's matchmaking, Elizabeth fixed her gaze on Alistair, encouraging him to discuss his goals and future aspirations. Alistair assumed center stage, alluding to his accomplishments with mathematics, finance, and banking in general. It was clear that he intended to climb the banking corporate ladder quickly, amassing wealth. He noted his desire to establish a foundation aimed at improving education, perhaps endowing a professorship in the arts in concert with this father. His boundless enthusiasm and animation captivated the table.

Charles then spoke.

"Alistair, there are six Harvard graduates here tonight," he noted, eyes fixated on the young financier. "Annette is also here, a current student in classics at Harvard Annex. And Alfred, an 1883 graduate of our medical school, intends to improve the health of our residents by establishing a hospital in Waltham, our neighboring city. We embrace all fields at Harvard, from the arts to the sciences. I certainly applaud your goal to support an endowed professorship in the arts, one perhaps emulating Stubby's professorship in English."

Stubby, while nodding in agreement, noted that his professorship was not endowed, in contrast to the proposal for the arts. Wincing slightly from the pinch on his leg from Ellen, Stubby returned to his soup, looking forward to the main dish.

"Alistair and Matthew, let us meet later this week to explore your ideas more thoroughly," said Charles in a manner bringing closure to the subject. Deferred to as dominant in the conversation, Charles's voice was that of power.

Interrupting the tone in the room, Annette cleared her voice, raising a question: "What, President Eliot, are your plans for admitting women to Harvard directly?"

"Women at Harvard," Charles repeated. As soup bowls were removed, replaced with slow-simmered roast beef cooked with onions, garlic, potatoes, and carrots and baked in individual flaky pies, Charles looked blankly at his plate, wishing for a reprieve from responding. His scowl at Amos did not silence Annette. Ever a politician, he glanced at Elizabeth, as if beseeching her to answer Annette's question.

"Annette, what a wonderful question. Let's hold on responding until everyone has been served our main dish," encouraged Elizabeth.

The individual roast beef pies were breathtaking, with strong, spicy aromas of beef mixed with butter, brandy, and cider. The aroma suffused the room, with guests anxious to taste their pies, the accompanying caramelized corn with fresh mint, and pear marmalade and soft French bread. With Bordeaux red wine paired with the main course, Elizabeth believed her guests would become increasingly comfortable, and more loquacious, as the dinner progressed.

As her guests began to enjoy their main course, Elizabeth returned to Annette's question.

"Charles," Elizabeth said, "at the Annex we discuss women's right to education, their need and desire to contribute to society, beyond homemaking and childcare. Perhaps you can provide your views on education for women. This is an excellent venue to share your thoughts."

Annette sought Charles's gaze, locking on his eyes without blinking.

"When I was inaugurated president in 1869, I claimed that the world knew next to nothing about the natural mental capacities of the female sex. Now, years later, I can say that I know more. I know that women's academic performance is stellar, their grit for learning substantial, and their passion for education immense. With civil freedom and social equality, women's roles in society can be limitless." Charles provided guests with a snapshot of steps he had taken at Harvard since assuming the presidency. He noted the Harvard Annex, with Harvard's professors serving as faculty for Annex students. He described future steps, most immediately to charter the Annex as a degree-granting institution within the commonwealth, to create a sister institution for women within the Harvard community.

Sipping his wine, Charles leaned across the table, speaking to Annette as if they were the only two in the room. "Annette, you may soon graduate from the institution I describe here today. You may be in the first class graduating from Harvard's sister institution."

Elizabeth added that she and Charles held regular meetings on this very subject and intended to bring closure to this matter soon.

Charles, stabbing a small bite of beef with his fork, noted that it was of paramount importance that Harvard admit women.

"It is simply time to do so," he concluded.

"Perhaps men and women will someday learn together in a united institution, but now we will begin the incremental process by advocating a sister institution."

"Thank you, Charles," said Elizabeth, smiling broadly.

"Well," said Elizabeth in a senatorial voice, "let us now hear from you, Alfred. Tell us about the hospital you are establishing in Waltham, and the Training School for Nurses associated with it. Do students at the school receive degrees upon graduation?" Elizabeth recognized Charles's admiration for Alfred, whom he considered a progressive, industrious Harvard alumni. Charles's maternal grandfather, Theodore Lyman, had been a successful Boston merchant with a summer home in Waltham, referred to as The Vale. Both Charles and Alfred loved Waltham, a city that bound them beyond the ties of Harvard.

Charles found medicine to be engaging, admixing skills in both sciences and arts. His appreciation for medicine, fueled by loss of his first wife and the mental distress of his son, galvanized his desire to transform Harvard's medical school into the nation's leading health care college. Horrified by Louis Agassiz's characterization of the medical school's exam period as rather "like the mad tea party in *Alice in Wonderland*," Charles had facilitated dramatic change in the program's curriculum as early as 1871. Alfred was Charles's young protégé. His dogged work in home care, complemented by his warm-hearted devotion to patients, inspired Charles to attend more vigorously to health education at the university. Uncharacteristically, Charles participated in fundraising activities associated with Alfred's hospital-building campaigns and events at the nursing school.

Alfred first thanked Elizabeth for her invitation to dinner and nodded his gratitude to Charles. As he spoke, Alfred focused on Annette, speaking to all as if through her. He thought her beautiful. A quiet family practice doctor, Alfred gravitated to her kind smile and wide-open, intelligent eyes.

Confident, Alfred captivated the table. He described milk stations located at key Waltham intersections for women to purchase milk for children at low cost, a health dispensary housed in the Charles Street Watch Company for treatment of employees' work injuries, home or hospital treatment of tuberculosis and other infections, new management of obstetrical emergencies, care of the dying, and other matters.

Alfred closed his summary with details on the Waltham Training School for Nurses together with the Waltham Hospital, both initially established in 1885. Nursing and medicine, to Alfred, were an inviolate team, a team necessary for the health of individuals and the larger community.

"Soon, a new, separate building for Waltham Hospital will open," Alfred noted. "This will mark the date when the hospital and the school will have separate buildings, each with independent administrations."

"I urge each of you," Alfred said, "to encourage young women to become nurses, to care for patients and families, and to help keep health our goal, not simply the construction of hospitals. Nurses are key to health. Their training must occur in colleges, with a defined curriculum, as occurs in medicine."

His calm but passionate summary concluded, Alfred stressed that "Doctors are needed, but more importantly, we need trained nurses for both community and hospital needs. The new Waltham Hospital will survive only if nurse training thrives."

Again, the room was quiet. Were guests expected to respond? Did Alfred have a request?

Annette again broke the silence. "Dr. Worcester, are you suggesting that Harvard educate nurses?"

Caught off guard by the bluntness of her question, Alfred regained his composure. "Yes," he replied, "Harvard must offer education for nursing, as it does for medicine and dentistry."

"Indeed," Alfred expanded, "my intent was to update you on health needs of our larger community and to invite you to participate in meeting these needs in any way reasonable."

Elizabeth sensed it was time to bring such discussions to a close and allow Caroline's plans for the evening to proceed as she had wished.

"Thank you, Alfred, for introducing us to both the Waltham Hospital and the Training School for Nurses. Your advocacy of college training for nursing is clear. This is a topic that we — Charles and I — will continue discussing in our regular meetings."

Elizabeth summoned the kitchen maids to serve dessert as guests continued to talk amongst themselves. Lemon syllabub — a light, creamy parfait of cream, sugar, and lemon juice, flavored generously with white wine and garnished with mint, nutmeg, and a slice of lemon — was a delectable ending to Elizabeth's memorable dinner.

"A marvelous evening!" Elizabeth told her guests as dessert was served. "So much to consider, future actions to undertake." With that, Elizabeth ushered her guests back to the parlor for light pastries and liqueurs. Guests grouped together according to their interests, with Annette, Alistair, and Alfred adjourning to

Elizabeth's back porch, sitting on the spacious wooden rocking chairs. Given Annette's interest in the Waltham hospital and training school, Alfred invited her to tour both sometime in the near future. Annette agreed to do so, and they set a date for the tour in the following week, after her classics mid-term examinations.

Now alone, Annette and Alistair relaxed. She smoked her cigarette with mouthpiece, coughing a bit less spastically with each draw as she got the knack of this new sin, and Alistair inhaled deeply on his Cuban cigar from Ybor City.

"We are a pair, aren't we?" queried Alistair.

"Yes, we are," Annette said quietly.

"Annette, I am not the type of man your mother wishes you to marry." Alistair looked directly at her.

"I sensed that might be so. I think that we can be wonderful friends." She smiled, continuing to rock in her chair.

Alistair, now safe, felt comfortable in their shared understanding. He made an impetuous invitation.

"Annette, there will be a Columbian Exhibition in a few months in Chicago, a World's Fair with many programs planned. Would you like to attend with me? It will be held for several months, so we could attend during your vacation from the Annex."

Charmed by his unconventionality, she accepted.

At home that evening, Annette reviewed events of the dinner party. My life is becoming charmingly complex, she thought, much as did Aphrodite's. Wondering if she would win the gold apple for being the fairest, Annette slept.

Confusion

"**S**top!"

Exasperated, with head buried in arms folded on her desk, Annette spoke to her mother without glancing at her.

"Mother, *please* understand!" Annette, her voice softening, turned to her mother. Arranged systematically on the floor around her desk lay Xenophon's *Anabasis*, Aeschylus's *Oresteia* trilogy, several Platonic dialogues, and the *Aeneid*, each with scrapes of paper marking specific sections. Disheartened by her mother's insistence that she shop for new clothing to favorably impress suitors, particularly Alistair, Annette frowned disdainfully at the fashion drawings Caroline brandished.

How could her mother be so unaware of the coursework she was studying at the Annex? Now in her third year toward a certificate in classics, Annette would be awarded a Bachelor of Arts degree at the completion of her fourth year if the Annex had the authority to grant degrees. Given the conversation at Elizabeth Agassiz's home recently, however, Annette was tentatively hopeful that the Annex would soon be granted the authority to award degrees, should it be named Harvard University's sister institution.

Drifting in thought, Annette glanced at Elizabeth Agassiz's leather-bound journal on her desk under Francis Allinson's *Greek Prose Composition Exercises for Writing*, one of her study guides for her exams. Elizabeth's journal was key to understanding the Annex's history, as well as roles that she and Charles Eliot played in framing it. I must review Elizabeth's journal soon, Annette thought.

Caroline, now on the edge of Annette's bed, demanded attention.

Annette had never seen her mother as agitated and annoyed as she was right now.

"Tomorrow, Mother, tomorrow. In one day, I begin my examinations in Greek and Latin. I have worked hard on these subjects. I intend to do very well." Feeling herself flush, Annette returned to the book opened on her desk, anticipating that her mother would leave.

Caroline continued, ignoring the cue.

"You will do well, Annie. All you do is study."

As she spoke, Annette began to appreciate the extent to which her mother was truly aghast by her shorter day dresses and bloomers, mirroring her strides toward independence. Caroline hoped to replace her daughter's new woman cycling costume, including bifurcated bloomers and shortened dresses, with more fashionable, stylish day dresses. What does a lady's wardrobe, her mother reminded her, say about the lady? Mother, Annette thought to herself, had become intentionally deaf.

"Your clothing," Caroline continued, "defines you. Your morning, afternoon, and evening wear must meet your station in our society." Hoping to dissuade Annette from the tawdry image of the Gibson Girl fad sweeping the country, Caroline said that a known seamstress would be hired to produce new clothing for Annette.

"And," Caroline added, reminding her daughter of promises made at the conclusion of Elizabeth's recent dinner, "your clothing must be appropriate to tour hospitals with doctors, attend a World's Fair with friends, or join a suitor for dinners and dancing. You do not want to be the focus of gossip."

Was Caroline concerned solely with Annette's attire, or, more likely, with what it represented? Did her daughter's appearance embarrass her? Had Caroline connected bloomers with a new woman's movement, one that would change women's lives forever? A fundamental change in women's roles in the Back Bay might spill over, irrevocably affecting Caroline herself.

"Let's return to this conversation after my exams are complete," offered Annette, attempting a conciliation that would get her mother out of her room.

While Caroline did not have the measurements and color preferences she sought, she was placated by her daughter's parting words.

Annette returned to the *Anabasis*.

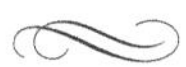

Normally quick to dismiss unwanted thoughts, Annette admitted feeling rattled by her mother's priorities, rendering her unable to focus clearly on her studies. She was also unnerved by her father's recent comments about President Eliot's lauded articles on the *new* education in *The Atlantic Monthly*, published twenty-three years earlier. Her father ranged through time, fishing for ideas to fuel his *Globe* and *Times* articles.

Both parents were aware of change in post-Civil War America, one fearful, the other excited. Knowing that she could manage her mother's fear, Annette set aside Xenophon to think about her father's embrace of Eliot's radical call for educational relevance.

Amos had kept copies of Eliot's articles, preserving them in a large gummed envelope further secured with a wax seal, symbolizing their value. Annette's father had given her the sealed envelope shortly after Elizabeth's dinner, counseling her to review the articles when she had the time to do so.

"Annie," Amos had said with reverence, "Charles is changing education in America. What he writes in these articles paves the way for American greatness."

With the *Anabasis* pushed to the side, Annette decided to read Eliot's articles. She knew she had a role to play in reading them. Her father, a writer emphasizing future rather than past, had recognized her own need as a woman to defend the utility of a college education. What was a given for men, he knew, required justification for women. She left her desk, propped two pillows on her bed, slipped her ivory-carved letter opener — a gift from her father — beneath the seal of her father's envelope, and began to read the February 1869 article. She devoured it first, paced around her room for a few minutes, and then resettled on her bed, the March 1869 article laid out in front of her.

Imaging herself a young woman in 1869, four years after Robert E. Lee surrendered to Ulysses S. Grant in Appomattox, Annette conjured images of a country still dangerously fragmented, with a tattered economy and destroyed cities. She closed her eyes.

Charles Eliot, Annette thought, saw opportunity in the desperation of post-Civil War America. To not only rebuild as a country, but also to advance as a world leader, America needed to change its educational system in radical ways. Characterizing education in the mid-nineteenth century as insufficient for a modern world, Eliot proposed a series of innovations based on pure and applied sciences, the living European languages, and mathematics. He also encouraged apprenticeships and practical laboratory benchwork, while at the same time advocating less emphasis on Latin and Greek.

Success in such a new system of education, Annette appreciated, would be highly dependent on revision of programs offered in preparatory schools. As Eliot had noted, preliminary schools are, in fact, what colleges make them. Thus, for students to graduate from a college program reorganized along the lines Eliot proposed, preparatory schools would need to provide expanded, enriched, and more diverse programs. Charles Eliot advocated alignment of education to the changing demands of American society. Advising Americans to "help freedom by judicious education," Eliot aimed to assure America's lead position among industrial nations.

Annette wondered if the editor had placed John Greenleaf Whittier's "Howard at Atlanta," a poem describing a conversation between a Union general and a Black schoolchild, as a message to readers. The phrase spoken by the child, "General, tell 'em we are rising" spoke across time. She could almost hear the child's voice.

Annette opened her eyes, returning to 1892.

Here is hope, she thought, enthusiastically. The issue is bigger than college education for women. Education itself must change. My role will be to figure just how I can play my part in this story.

If Eliot is correct, Annette thought, then is my program of study in the classics questionable? Pacing again, Annette sought to calm her racing mind. Eliot espoused broadened education, with sciences, arts, medicine, and other fields to be offered, thus fueling economic growth and prosperity after the devastation of civil war. While he had not denied the value of the classics, he had pleaded for additional courses in specialized education, requiring reduction in mandatory courses in Greek and Latin. All the seven sister colleges, named for the Greek Pleiades, daughters of Atlas and Pleione, were famed for education in the classics, with the Harvard Annex promoting the excellence of its Harvard faculty.

I am a classist. I have become arcane, she thought, and I am proud of the force of that.

Annette wondered if college education was shifting too radically toward practicality at the expense of knowledge of the ancient world. She understood the arguments for embracing the modern, but she also wondered if those making them understood the losses. Her mental discipline and tenacity, she believed, could be attributed to her attention to the textual translation, along with her sharp skills in memory, reasoning, analysis, and discrimination.

And, while she thought these fine outcomes, she also acknowledged that they were not necessarily lucrative. Annette understood that her employment options were limited when she completed her master's degree. Teach Latin, perhaps some Greek, in a girls' school, such as Arthur Gilman's Cambridge School, or become a wife, mother, and homemaker, or, as she defined it, an educated domestic servant.

Subjugating unsettling thoughts to pass her upcoming exams with high honors, Annette focused, holding confusion for another day.

Too excited now for Xenophon's history, she turned to the *Aeneid* and its vibrancy as the founding story of Rome. Uncertainty ebbed quickly as she began her translation of the *Aeneid*, one task of the examination. Taking the role of emperor in 27 BC after the assassination of his great uncle, Julius Caesar, Augustus had restored order to Rome, creating a political, military, and economic empire that lasted just over fourteen hundred years until the fall of Constantinople. Commissioned to write a poem of the founding of the empire by Augustus himself, Virgil wrote the *Aeneid* during the last years of his life. Annette liked to think that the *Aeneid* linked the world of ancient Greece, described in Homer's *Iliad* and *Odyssey*, with the world of Rome. As she translated, she thought of the line by Edgar Allen Poe in "To Helen" describing "the glory that was Greece / And the grandeur that was Rome."

She thought of Virgil as the thread connecting both civilizations. Origin stories, she knew, were important.

The passage to be translated was from Book VI, the last one hundred and fifty lines describing the descent of Aeneas to the underworld. There, his father, Anchises, shows him the world that is yet to be. Annette recalled that Aeneas had carried the old man out of Troy on his back as the city burned, and that burning was the beginning of the founding of Rome. In destruction was the beginning.

Before she began her translation, she looked quickly to the end for her favorite lines:

> *Anchises natum per singula duxit*
> *e animum famae venientis amore,*
> *exim bella viro memorat quae deinde gerenda*

She recalled John Dryden's translation:

> *Which when Anchises to his son had shown,*
> *And fir'd his mind to mount the promis'd throne,*
> *He tells the future wars, ordain'd by fate.*

That was it, she thought: *incenditque animum famae venientis amore.* Set fire to his heart with the coming love of fame. So much rested on the genitive form of the participle *venientis.* So much rested on coming.

Annette was aware of Virgil's dactylic hexameters, the poetic form he had used in each of the twelve books of the poem. And she knew that Dryden had transformed that form into closed couplets. She would not try either but decided, instead, to use heightened prose. She tried out her favorite line quickly on a separate sheet of paper:

> *Anchises led his son, Aeneas, over every scene, setting fire to his son's soul, with longing for the glory that was yet to be. Anchises then tells of the wars that the hero next must wage.*

Contemporary and connected, she thought, with focused illustration of pronoun references, and a little flourish for emphasis. Our world improved by theirs.

This, she thought, would do nicely. She placed a sheet of paper just below the palm of her left hand in order not to smudge the ink. Sinister, she thought, and smiled as she began.

I could do this forever, she thought. The sheer joy of the solitary work, the peacefulness of translation, and the superb clarity of thought associated with translation were giddying to her. Proud of her knowledge, she temporarily put aside questions of utility, larger questions of contributions to society. For now, she was convinced that honors in the classics would be hers. Utility and contribution would be considered thereafter.

As the sun set, Annette reviewed the rules for cases in Greek prose composition. She rehearsed tense and voice, pronouns and the genitive absolute, the dative case, temporal clauses, and specialized vocabulary. Spending hours on translating required

Greek passages from Homer and Herodotus, as well as Latin passages from Cicero and Virgil, Annette familiarized herself with questions on the usual forms and constructions of the languages and on prosody. She had to work harder on Greek than on Latin. She often dreamt in Latin but never in Greek.

To gain additional practice so that she could move fluidly from English to both Greek and Latin, she translated short passages from her father's books. In 1890, Amos published *Midnight Talks at the Club*, a collection of papers originally printed in Sunday issues of *The New York Times*, where he was then an editorial writer. Only one year later, he published *Beyond the Bourn*, narrated by a person visiting a planet where an ideal anarchy had stimulated rapid artistic and scientific advancement. Annette's final exercise, after eight continuous hours of study, was translation of the prefatory notes in each of her father's books to both languages.

Annette thoroughly enjoyed her father's books and editorials, provocative writing that lifted her beyond the commonplace. He was thoughtful and deliberative. She was always complimented when her mother, frustrated with Annette's lack of kitchen skills, compared her to Amos. Stacking her books on her desk, Annette glanced at Elizabeth's journal, Eliot's *Atlantic Monthly* articles, and her father's books neatly arranged on the windowsill apron, itself serving as a bookshelf.

She reached for a cigarette in her pocket and headed for the gazebo. She always knew when a good day's work had been done.

As expected, within a week, Annette found that she had performed exceedingly well on her examinations, achieving the highest scores in her class. Since her visit with Alfred to the Waltham hospital and school was two weeks away, she decided to first organize the next meeting of the Annex book club, with Elizabeth Agassiz as guest.

Annette knew the meeting would be unusual. Rarely does a school president attend student book club meetings, oftentimes considered by administrators as social rather than scholarly events. Annette posted the date, time, and place of the meeting on the bulletin board reserved for student communications outside the main student parlor in Fay House. The topic, *Elizabeth Agassiz and the Establishment of the Society for the Collegiate Instruction of Women*, intrigued students, with attendance expected to be greater than the room's capacity.

At Elizabeth's request, the book club meeting was held at Alice Mary Longfellow's home on Brattle Street, a short walk of about two minutes from Fay House. Alice's home, built in 1759 and employed by General George Washington as headquarters of the Continental Army from 1775 to 1776, was Georgian in style, with two floors, each with four identical rooms. It was spacious with large windows and beautiful landscaping. Due to Alice's gracious generosity, Longfellow House was the frequent site of Annex meetings.

Daughter of Henry Wadsworth Longfellow, Alice, at twenty-eight years old, had been appointed in 1879 to the Society, a group of seven women and one man, Arthur Gilman. As a special student at the Harvard Annex from 1879 to 1881, and again from 1884 to 1890, Alice was a fervent supporter of the Annex and women's education. Considered a conservative silent suffragist, she frequently participated in women's causes, often opening her home for meetings of women's clubs. Her association with Elizabeth and the Annex for over twelve years was a great source of pride for Alice, now eager to participate in the Annex's book club.

At forty-two, Alice was youthful and fragile in appearance, with dark-blue eyes in an oval face framed by wavy graying brown hair swept up in braids held in place by a thin rose-colored diadem. Wearing a fashionable cranberry-colored dress with tight bodice and high lacy collar, Alice quietly held the attention of people in her presence. With inherited wealth from her father, Alice never married, but did enjoy a long relationship with Fanny Stone, whose portrait hung prominently in a first-floor guest parlor room.

The club meeting began as scheduled at 7:00 pm.

Eighteen students, Annette, Elizabeth, and Alice formed a circle with their chairs, Annette serving as meeting convenor.

Dressed in short dress and bloomers, Annette was interrupted in her introductions as her aunt, Ellen, entered the parlor with a flourish.

"Excuse my lateness. My husband, Francis, required my assistance in his library, so please be annoyed at him, not me," Ellen said with a coy smile. The group accommodated Ellen, enlarging their circle to allow her to sit by her niece. Ellen casually squeezed Annette's hand, saying "please continue."

"Our President Agassiz needs no introduction, but I do wish to tell you about my possession of her journal."

Annette carefully removed Elizabeth's leather-bound journal from her bookbag, loosening the thin straps that tied it. Asking each person to hold the journal without opening it, Annette said that Elizabeth had requested that she review its contents and bring it to the meeting for discussion.

"This journal is a legacy. It documents a courageous female leader's role in the education of women in our country. It is humbling. It must be preserved for its historical significance." Looking at Elizabeth, Annette requested that she tell her story, beginning with the establishment of a school for girls in her home in Cambridge in 1859.

When her journal made its way to her, Elizabeth began her story. Clearing her throat, she first asked the group to call her Lizzie, a nickname given to her by her family and used by her friends.

"I consider you all friends, champions of women's causes." Elizabeth began with her marriage to Louis, a renowned biologist, geologist, and professor at Harvard University. When her family needed additional income to supplement her husband's travel and other work-related expenses, she established a school for girls in their Cambridge home. This school was a pioneering effort in women's education, remaining active from 1855 to 1863. When her husband died in 1873, Elizabeth remained in Cambridge, continuing to enjoy the company of her Harvard acquaintances, many of whom had been invited to her gatherings during her husband's tenure at the university.

One person, Arthur Gilman, became a lifelong friend and colleague to Elizabeth.

"Arthur loved his daughter. He refused to send her either to Vassar or Wellesley, women's colleges in which most of the faculty were not educated at Harvard, Princeton, or Yale, let alone Oxford or Cambridge." Arthur, Elizabeth stressed with an arched brow, would not tolerate second-rate education for his daughter. He approached President Eliot at Harvard, recommending that the university become competitive with other colleges and develop a plan for the education of women. Together, Arthur and Charles mapped out a staged plan, beginning with the establishment of an executive group of women to recruit Harvard classics faculty on a part-time basis. Once recruited, these faculty would instruct women in Cambridge and Boston in rooms rented on Appian Way.

The Private Collegiate Instruction for Women, with Elizabeth appointed as president, was formally established in 1879.

Elizabeth, retrieving a circular dated February 22, 1879, from her journal, slowly read the following faded statements handwritten on it:

"A number of professors and other instructors at Harvard College have consented to give private tuition to properly qualified young women who desire to pursue advanced courses of study in Cambridge. Other professors, whose occupations prevent them from giving such tuition, are willing to assist young women by giving advice and by lectures. No instruction will be provided of a lower grade than that given in Harvard College." Elizabeth returned the circular to her journal. "Thus," she said to the delight of the room, "mountains come to Mohammed."

Forty-four Harvard faculty participated in the program, soon commonly referred to as the Harvard Annex. Elizabeth indicated that the Annex, a quick success, was incorporated as the Society for the Collegiate Instruction of Women in 1882, offering fifty-one courses in thirteen subject areas.

Turning to Alice Longfellow, Elizabeth thanked her for her long-standing support of the Annex, noting that the next stage in the campaign for women's collegiate education would be the chartering of the Annex as degree-granting, a sister institution to Harvard.

While Arthur Gilman was not present, Elizabeth thanked him also, noting, with a soft reverence in her voice, that "his original drive for excellence and equality propelled our movement. He continues to serve as the secretary for the Annex, even after he established the Cambridge School for Girls in 1886 as a feeder school for the Annex." Just as Charles had claimed in his 1869

Atlantic articles, Elizabeth and Arthur were keenly aware that collegiate education must be based on a strong academic base. Annette understood that her current success in the classics at the Annex was partly attributable to her attendance at the Cambridge School.

"What will you do now with your journal, Elizabeth?" asked Ellen.

Elizabeth looked to Annette and said that she and her pupil had a plan.

Annette, glancing at Elizabeth as if on cue, responded.

Fearing that she might misspeak, Annette read a statement she had previously drafted together with Elizabeth and Ellen. Everyone knew that this part of the meeting had been carefully staged and that there was a bond among the three women.

"Harvard instituted the archives as a separate unit of the university library in 1851, over forty years ago. The archives is a natural home for Elizabeth's journal, including personal communications, circulars, incorporation documents, correspondence, and more."

"Lizzie, as we will now call you," Annette continued, "represents the Annex's early history, the forerunner to any future sister institution to Harvard. It seems appropriate and reasonable that her materials would be collected, cataloged, and placed in special charge of the university."

As Ellen posed the question of the journal's fate, Alice had motioned for the household staff to bring forward trays of Asti Spumante, freshly poured and sparkling. Annette raised her glass first and gave the toast.

"Here's to Lizzie."

After a moment of silence, the students stood up and cheered, rushing up on Elizabeth and shaking her hand. The timing had been perfect.

Alice ushered her guests into a second parlor, one arranged for late evening tea and shortbread cookies. Over sips and bites, Elizabeth told Annette that she had a meeting scheduled with President Eliot the next day. Inviting Annette to join the meeting, Elizabeth requested that she inform the president of their proposal to archive the leather-bound journal in the university archives. Aware of the honor of being in the room in the first place, Annette accepted the invitation.

After details for the next day were finalized, Elizabeth and Annette turned their attention to Alice and the other guests. Several students had asked Alice to reveal her favorite poems written by her father. She said that his poem "The Children's Hour," written in 1863 when she was thirteen years old, was her favorite. Reminding her of the caretaker role for her younger sisters that she assumed after her mother's death two years earlier, she believed that his description of her as "grave Alice" in the poem was accurate and appropriate.

"My mother," said Alice, "thought me impetuous and full of character and originality." She claimed that after her mother's death, her former impetuous character was dulled by daily tasks, although she did enjoy vacations for many years with her father. Her mother's estate willed to her at death ensured Alice financial independence and freedom for life. She neither wanted nor needed to marry.

"I am aligned to women, and to women's causes, particularly the Annex. I hope to host many more events for the Annex, including graduation ceremonies."

As guests left Longfellow House, Annette was joyous. If we remain in solidarity, then change can happen, she thought. She recalled Virgil: *Audentes fortuna iuvat*. If fortune did indeed favor the brave, then no braver women could be found then Ellen, Lizzie, and Alice.

Counting the book club meeting a major success, Annette turned her thoughts to Alfred Worcester, his hospital, and the training school for nurses. I need to understand the role of nurses, and how nurses are educated, prior to touring with him. Having never been ill, apart from brief bouts of congestion, runny nose, and coughing in winter, illness was alien to Annette. Ever competitive, she was determined to become familiar with the most common diseases prevalent in Massachusetts prior to visiting his facilities. She would work up the diseases and their definitions just as she worked up ancient vocabulary, one word at a time.

Annette was both intrigued and perplexed by Alfred Worcester. At Elizabeth Agassiz's recent dinner party, Alfred Worcester had spoken of his heavy patient workload, frequent home care visits, and the exhausting burden of keeping up with advances in science. He was also clearly thrilled by his work in medicine. Passionate about the field of bacteriology, Alfred had spoken with great excitement about Robert Koch's discovery of the bacterium causing tuberculosis, an infectious disease best understood within the evolving germ theory of disease. Annette was charmed that, as Alfred warmed to his subject, he was unaware of the mess he was making as pastry crumbs tumbled around his chair.

The trip from Annette's family home at 1564 Massachusetts Avenue in Cambridge to Cutler House, home of the hospital and school, took a little over thirty minutes on cobblestone roads. Rising early, Annette had looked forward to the day of the meeting and donned what was now becoming her short dress and bloomers uniform. The morning was brilliant and sunny, and Alfred greeted her on the front porch of the house. Deciding on a no-nonsense approach, she got to the point.

"Dr. Worcester, you are a busy doctor. Why are you taking precious time to show me the hospital and school?"

"Miasma, or night air as my family had called it, does not cause tuberculosis."

How had he gotten from her question to that answer? She paused for a moment, both perplexed and amused.

Tuberculosis, Alfred continued, was caused by a bacterium, calling for improved personal cleanliness and organized sanitary measures, particularly important in cities.

Annette wondered how she fit into his thinking. Surely, he could not believe she had a role in nursing. Surely, she thought, he understands that I am a student in the classics.

She hoped his thoughts would slow down enough for her to get on the train in his mind.

"Annette, William Sedgwick, a professor of sanitary science and public health at the Massachusetts Institute of Technology, said that *before* 1880, we knew nothing, but *after* 1890, *we knew it all*. This has been a glorious ten years." He had difficulty containing his excitement. "We are on the very brink of great change in disease management!"

His tone suddenly shifted as he added that "nothing will change, however, if there aren't enough educated doctors and nurses to fight disease, and more importantly, help people stay well."

Annette decided it would be best, at least for her, to hold further questions, and to simply wait for Alfred to unravel his story as they toured the house. Perhaps, she thought, his excitement overwhelms his thinking, making it difficult for him to converse.

Alfred motioned to a large sign with deep-red letters bordered by gold margins: *The Waltham Hospital and Training School for Nurses.* He told Annette that the house was owned by Dr. Edward Cutler on Main Street in Waltham, currently also housing his friends, the Frank Christmas family.

Alfred said that Edward Cutler, one of the oldest physicians in the city, had long cherished the idea that a hospital for the relief of distress and illness would be established in Waltham. According to Alfred, Cutler offered his home as both a hospital and training school in 1885, with four rooms for patients and the rest of the house for the school, as well as members of the Frank Christmas family, close allies of the school. As needs of both the hospital and school expanded, the building was renovated to accommodate fifteen ward beds and two cribs. Shortly thereafter, Cutler relocated the Christmas family to a new home, enabling more space to accommodate boarding all pupil nurses.

Listening carefully but remaining flummoxed, Annette frowned, wondering where the improbably named Christmas family fit in to all of this. She decided to venture a question.

"For exactly how many years has the Cutler house been a working hospital and school?"

Suddenly, Alfred seemed to realize how far afield he had gone from Annette's initial question. He knew he needed to slow down.

"I apologize, Annette," he said. "Yes, in March of 1886, the Cutler home was incorporated as the Waltham Hospital, also known as the Cutler Hospital by residents, and the Waltham Training School for Nurses. In 1887, the house was renovated, as I mentioned previously, with space for more ward beds and cribs. Please bear with me. Let me tell you about our hospital and school, and some of the key changes in public health and medicine that have created wonderful opportunities."

Our worlds are so different, Alfred thought. Escorting her to the spacious front veranda of the white house, Alfred gestured for Annette to join him in sculpted wooden rocking chairs. Before retelling the brief history of the building, however, he placed the training school's silver graduation pin in her hand, the engraved motto *fides, spes.*

"Latin for faith and hope," Annette translated, before Alfred could do so. "Quite a lovely aphorism for a school."

"I had forgotten how proficient you are in the classics. I am sure your Latin is *much* better than mine." Alfred was animated again, pleased to talk with someone knowledgeable in the classics *and* interested, perhaps, in medicine.

"I initially failed in my Greek admission test at Harvard, needing an additional year in preparation. When I was accepted in 1874, I worried that perhaps a mistake had been made, and that I would never graduate from medical school. Fortunately, I did graduate in 1883, despite my abysmal knowledge of the classics. But I am blathering now and must return to the story of our hospital and school."

"Annette, our patients desperately need nurses. They need more than night watchers, friendly visitors, or even physicians. They need better than the dissolute, drunken Sairey Gamp in Dickens' novel *Martin Chuzzlewit.* They need educated nurses, trained in returning patients to health, in working with doctors to manage illness, and in promoting sanitary science. You are an educated young woman." Alfred ceased pacing and faced her, hands pushed forcibly into his coat pockets. He trained his piercing blue eyes directly on her.

"I invited you here to help me answer a question: how can our school attract young women to the field of nursing today?" There, thought Alfred, I have said it. I need women like you, he thought. It may well be, he continued, that I need you.

"Tell me more," replied Annette. She was getting the knack of him. He was forever *in medias res*, and she needed to get him to slow the train in his mind just enough for her to hop onboard.

Her question was answered, and, as if delivering a prepared speech, Alfred finally relaxed in a rocking chair. Hands placed lightly on armrests, he now described Waltham.

Transformed by industries in mid-century, the city of Waltham moved away from farming to a busy mix of factories and crowded housing. Tuberculosis, syphilis, work injuries, and malnutrition overwhelmed Waltham's dispensaries for the poor. Paying patients faced challenges in securing private-duty nurses for home care and doctors for home visits. Even pest houses for infectious cases and almshouses, or asylums, built for health care of the indigent, became overburdened. Families had gradually become unable to care for their acutely sick members.

"Hospitals," Alfred stressed, "do not replace families in caring for the sick. But they do follow scientific principles of cleanliness and sanitation."

"Annette, have you heard of Florence Nightingale?" Alfred, leaning forward in his chair toward her, waited for her reply.

"Yes, I have heard the name, but I know little of her," Annette said, interested to hear his description of her.

Alfred, smiling, was now in his element. As he stretched his long legs out before him, he explained that hospitals evolved as science did, enabling severely ill patients to heal, given strict sanitary practices to control infection. Nightingale, a renowned statistician, hospital administrator, and nurse, served as Alfred's consultant when the school was designed in 1885. According to Alfred, Nightingale had described hospitals as a "hard necessity of an inferior and imperfect civilization — a place for proper care to be given if good care could not be given in the home." Proud of his relationship with Nightingale, Alfred said he followed her advice in the formation of the training school, with teachers providing experiences in both hospital care as well as home care nursing. Nurses manage hospital patients throughout the day, every day, while home visits are scheduled on a part-time basis.

"Commonly, Annette, hospitals are built first, with training schools to follow. Without pupils to provide daily patient care, there would be no need for hospitals. In our case, the school came first, necessitating a hospital for educational purposes as well as care for very sick patients." Alfred had taken Nightingale's lead, keeping strict statistics on patients, including age, gender, diagnosis, length of stay, and treating physician. He explained that his training at the Lying-In Hospital during his last year of medical school reinforced his demand for two essentials: complete patient records and data, and educated nurses. By the time he completed his rotation at the Lying-In Hospital, he had provided the nursing staff regular lectures in obstetrics, infectious diseases, and postpartum care.

"Our records demonstrate excellent outcomes," Alfred reported. The train was pulling from the station, and he stood.

"Since our doors opened in 1885, our beds have been full and our student enrollment has grown, with our graduates sought by many in the region. My colleagues and I, along with Miss Charlotte Macleod, our training school superintendent, want our pupils to be college educated. At our recent dinner at Miss Agassiz's home, President Eliot said the institution was moving toward enrolling women."

"I want more, and faster." Alfred began to pace on the porch.

"Like physicians and dentists, nurses must be college educated, with rotations to various patient services, in hospitals, homes, and other settings. Nurses cannot be simply trained; they must be educated to think, to make decisions, to teach health to the public." Pointing to himself, Alfred said that "doctors treat illness, nurses return patients and families to health, to self-sufficiency." Alfred returned to his rocking chair, thoughts adrift somewhere between the exhilaration of science and the complexities of care delivery. He was gone.

"I see," said Annette. She stood, leaning against the banister of the porch, facing Alfred so that he might focus.

"You have two requests as I understand it," she said. "First, you want my advice in promoting nursing as a viable field for young women to engage in. Second, you want to elicit my help in advocating for a Harvard School of Nursing. If the first goes well, you proceed to the second. Do I understand correctly?"

"Yes, you do," replied Alfred, without looking at her.

"Of course, you have my assistance on both counts. I too believe in education for women. I must ask one more question. Why have you taken this as your responsibility?"

"Nursing," replied Alfred, "and medicine are not separate professions. Nurses and doctors combine skills to care for patients.

We are responsible for each other. Doctors cannot simply escape from worrying about their patients because nurses are caring for them, nor can nurses provide care without cooperating with doctors. At present, I see training of nurses as part of my work. They, in turn, teach me, particularly so with home care. Remember also that nursing is now a respected field, one with employment opportunities that do not compete with those of men. I cannot practice medicine without working with nurses. It is truly that simple, Annette."

"As for you," he now looked at her again, "Lizzie says you are brilliant, and your aunt says you are awakening."

Suddenly, Annette realized that he had investigated her. He had spoken to Elizabeth, perhaps at Faye House, and must have had the chance to ask about her when dining with Uncle Stubby and Aunt Ellen. Her presence on the porch was no accident. She realized that women counted to this man.

"Well, please do let me see your hospital and school," Annette said, opening the door for him.

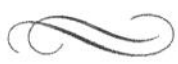

The sweeping porch encircling the lightly faded white, two-story colonial building was the most impressive feature of the Waltham Hospital and Training School for Nurses. Each of the four sections of the wide sunporch framing the square building offered several reclining and rocking chairs, each intended for tuberculosis patients to enjoy fresh air.

The dark mahogany doors that Alfred and Annette stepped through opened to a central hallway dividing the building into two areas, one side exclusive for private patients and the other for dormitory rooms, a classroom, a dining room, and a first-floor kitchen. Rooms designated for hospital use were large, with each patient room accommodating several patients, wardrobes for each, side chairs, overbed tables, and bedside stands complete with urinals and bedpans.

The dining room doubled as an operating room as needed.

A glass cabinet with three shelves holding surgical instruments, alcohol bottles, wash basins, and other surgical supplies stood next to a China hutch on one side of the mahogany dining table. In another corner, on the other side of the table, a large oak chest with hinged lid stored extra blankets, pillows, and sheets to be used when the room functioned as an operating theater. Above all else, the building was configured for practical use, every inch valuable for a particular function.

"You must be Miss Fiske," smiled Miss Charlotte Macleod, the superintendent of the training school, taking Annette's hand and shaking it firmly. Tall, exceptionally thin, with dark-brown hair worn unusually short and light-gray eyes just below perfect bangs, Miss Macleod wore a white nurse's apron with deep front pockets. She ushered Annette and Alfred into the central foyer, asking them if they would like tea and biscuits.

"When we first opened, an elderly Irishman who had broken a leg from falling while inebriated called me the *head lady*, a title that people still use today. Annette, please just call me Charlotte."

"Dr. Worcester has been eager to have you visit. A few months after I graduated from the Waltham School in June of 1891, I became the nursing superintendent. Since then, encouraged by Dr. Worcester, we at Waltham have discussed nursing as a profession requiring college education. I hear that you are a classics student at the Annex. Perhaps with your advice, we can find ways to attract college-educated young women to enroll in our school. Indeed, perhaps our school will someday convert to a college program."

Charlotte served Annette and Alfred tea and biscuits, reviewing the school's basic curriculum, rotations to the hospital and patient homes, and the roles of probationers, or probies as Charlotte called them, and pupil nurses.

Charlotte then circulated to patient rooms, introducing Annette to each patient. On the first floor, a thirty-two-year-old man was immobilized in bed with a leg fracture sustained while working at the Hood Rubber Company in Watertown, about three miles from Waltham. A pupil nurse was wrapping his leg wound in a cloth bandage, after which she would apply wooden splints on both sides of his leg to stabilize his limb. His roommate, an eighty-two-year-old man with a history of seizures, had recently fallen at home, hitting his head on a concrete stairway. His pupil nurse was examining his neurological status, looking at his pupils, checking the strength of his hand grasp, and asking him the date. The man was confused and experiencing frequent seizures, and his family questioned if he had the falling sickness demon, a dreaded mental sickness that would bring evil to his family. They sought relief at Waltham, believing that the famous Dr. Worcester could conjure a miracle cure.

Before Charlotte reached the second-floor patient rooms, a nervous probie interrupted her, hurriedly explaining that a young mother with consumption had been brought by her husband to the hospital for treatment. Emaciated and debilitated, with pale skin and deep dark circles under her eyes, the woman had been carried to the hospital in a carriage, wrapped in blankets. She incessantly coughed bloody sputum, complaining of chronic chest and back pain, and chronic fatigue.

Alfred, while holding the patient's hand, turned to her husband and explained that he would listen to her lungs before deciding if she could be treated at the hospital. Using his biaural stethoscope engraved with his initials—a medical school graduation gift from his family—Alfred listened to her lungs, both front and back.

Shaking his head slightly, Alfred spoke directly to the patient, telling her that her disease was too advanced for treatment at the Waltham Hospital. Gently, he recommended that she go home and rest in the company of her family. He instructed her husband to construct a waterbed for his wife, a bed-shaped box filled with water and covered by a rubber sheet firmly cemented to the box rims. "Such a waterbed will give your wife great comfort," he told her husband.

"Stay with your wife, sir. Your company now is the best treatment for her."

Alfred shook hands with the patient and her husband before rejoining Annette and Charlotte in the foyer.

"If he cannot, or won't, manage his wife, then he may bring her to a pest house, Annette," Charlotte explained. "Pestilence houses are places to quarantine patients with infectious diseases. There consumptives die. We try to convince people to allow sick family members to die at home rather than in a pest house." Charlotte was weary of tuberculosis, and eager to attempt any intervention with an outcome that did not include death.

"Charlotte," Alfred said, "I would like us to begin using the Carasso method to treat pulmonary tuberculosis patients here at our hospital. What do you think of this method?" For a few minutes, Charlotte and Alfred discussed the Carasso method, deciding to explore it further at the next hospital meeting. Understanding little,

Annette thought that this must be how her mother felt when she and her sister talked about foreign language translation at dinner.

"We have other patients on the second floor, one infant with diphtheria and one adult female with dysentery. While each is slowly recovering, we would prefer that they be treated elsewhere," said Alfred. "We cannot contain infectious diseases in our small hospital. And babies are particularly vulnerable to fluid loss and dehydration when infected. We will surely need a separate area for infectious diseases as well as a babies' unit soon. The pupil nurses have the primary responsibility to manage these patients, hydrate them, maintain their temperatures, prevent pneumonia, and ensure appropriate nutrition."

Alfred shifted attention to Annette, hopeful that she was neither bored nor disillusioned.

She was neither. He saw that her eyes were flashing.

"It appears that the probies have significant responsibility," Annette offered. "Are they taught anatomy and physiology? Disease mechanisms? Treatment options? Are lines drawn between functions of doctors and nurses? I would like to learn more about what pupil nurses are taught, along with the books they read, and the credentials of the faculty who teach them."

Annette had entered a new, and different, world. Intrigued by it, she and Alfred briefly discussed the need for both a baby unit and an infectious disease unit at Waltham Hospital as they prepared to leave for a home visit that Alfred felt she would benefit from. Saying her goodbyes to Charlotte Macleod and the pupil nurses and probies, Annette returned to the carriage, with Alfred taking the reins.

"Our first home visit will be to a young woman experiencing her first pregnancy. She is now early in her ninth month and is already reporting labor pains. She has high blood pressure and, although she is limiting her salt intake, I am worried about her. We have a seasoned pupil nurse on rotation to her home as well as a probie, so we'll be able to get a good picture of her pregnancy status." Alfred seemed distracted, and Annette found herself wondering about the young new mother-to-be and her future. How many children would she have? Her mother had only three children, an unusually small number given that most women had six to eight. Annette realized that chief among the many advantages of wealth was the ability to say no.

"Alfred, how frequently do mothers die during childbirth?" Linking death to childbirth, Annette was seeing family life as potentially dangerous for women.

"Women may die during delivery, or in the time immediately following it. When I was at the Lying-In Hospital, some died of hemorrhage, some of seizures, others from sepsis. High blood pressure seems to be the biggest problem, occasionally causing seizures and then death during delivery. The baby, in such cases, usually dies also. I have seen it a few times."

"It is," he paused as if searching for a word, "horrifying."

"If our patient, or her baby, is in distress, I will suggest a Caesarean section."

"Perhaps you know," said Annette, "that the word *Caesarean* comes from the Latin *caesus*, to cut. Julius Caesar was said to have been born by Caesarean section. In ancient times, mothers did not survive such procedures."

"Absolutely true," Alfred replied. "The Caesarean section was performed only to save the child. The mother died. Today, many doctors do craniotomies on fetuses that are wedged in the uterus, preventing descent. In those cases, the baby dies to save the mother. I would never perform that. Rather, I would plan a lower abdominal horizontal incision, open the uterus, and remove the baby, allowing both mother and baby to survive. I take my Greek Hippocratic Oath very seriously." Alfred recounted his few experiences with this procedure, noting that the uncertainty surrounding the surgery was daunting.

"Let's hope that our mother does not need surgery," said Alfred, making a cross on his chest. "If she does, then we'll have to bring her to the hospital. I don't have ether for anesthesia in my doctor's bag." Alfred indicated that neither the hospital nor his patient had telephones, thus they would transport her in their carriage if she needed surgery.

Alice, twenty-two years old and in her last month of pregnancy, lived in a third-floor two-room apartment in a tenement on Ash Street, neighboring the Waltham Watch Factory. As they approached Alice's address, Annette asked Alfred how he wished to explain her presence on the visit.

"I am recruiting you to our training school. Before making your decision, you wanted a realistic understanding of the role of the modern nurse. If Alice does not want you present, then you can retire to our carriage." Matter-of-fact and calm. An excellent answer, thought Annette. She wondered if he had done this with other women before.

A pupil nurse answered Alfred's door knock, looking relieved to see him. A tall girl with a robust figure, Betty, the pupil nurse, flushed with beads of sweat on her face, led them quietly to the patient's bed.

"I have been here for five hours with Alice. Her boyfriend, the father of her baby, has not been home. Alice's contractions have slowed, and I have not felt any fetal movements for the past hour, even when conducting Leopold's maneuvers. Her heart rate is increasing. I cannot hear the fetal heart with my ear to her abdomen. I think the baby may be in trouble." Betty stepped back, allowing Alfred to examine Alice.

Alice opened her eyes to Alfred's loud calling of her name, but she was otherwise nonresponsive. She did nothing when he listened to her lung sounds and abdomen, nor did she move when he palpated her abdomen.

"I fear the worst." Alfred hurriedly packed his doctor's bag and asked Betty to help him and the probie carry Alice down the stairs to the two-horse carriage. He held Alice in his arms while Betty kept Alice's head elevated and the probie held his elbow fast to help him down the stairs. Annette followed, offering to serve as driver of the coach. The woman, still wavering between conscious and unconscious as they reached the carriage, rested across Betty and Alfred, the probie holding tightly on the top of the carriage to steady herself. She ran to the hospital doors as soon as the carriage slowed, asking Charlotte Macleod to prepare the dining table as an operating suite.

All moved quickly. By the time she reached the table, Alice was unconscious with a blood pressure of 208/110.

"Eclampsia," said Alfred. "We can expect seizures now."

Alice's abdomen was prepared, lighting was increased, and the surgical supplies were arranged appropriately by Betty. Alfred put on an operating gown and mask, as did Betty. Charlotte and

Annette stood by as operating room assistants, to do whatever task was needed. Meanwhile, other pupil nurses prepared a bed for Alice and a cradle for the baby, assuming successful outcomes.

Alfred became a different man. The train had stopped dead. He was focused, assured. Each move was deliberate, executed with precision.

As Betty delivered ether anesthesia to Alice, Alfred held his scalpel in readiness. Once Alice was unconscious, Alfred incised her lower abdomen, made a horizontal cut, opened the uterus, cut the umbilical cord, and removed the baby, giving him to Charlotte. Charlotte rapidly removed fluid from the baby's mouth and upper airway, giving the baby boy a tap on his back to stimulate crying.

The boy gasped, then erupted into a hearty cry. Alfred and Betty worked simultaneously to maintain Alice's breathing and to repair her uterus and abdomen. Once her breathing was assured, non-laborious, and even, Alfred completed his surgical repair, placing a large sponge dressing over the wound.

Patient, baby, doctor, and nurse breathed with relief.

Betty handed the baby to Alice.

They had both lived.

The probies moved them both to their room, with the child in a cradle next to his mother.

Standing in the doorway of their room, Annette looked in on them, overwhelmed by the events of the last three hours. I must speak with Alfred before I leave, she thought. I cannot simply go home and return to translations. Might this Waltham world be mine someday?

Alfred, Betty, Charlotte, and the probie were in the kitchen, silently sipping tea.

"Join us," said Charlotte, pointing to an empty chair at the table.

Alfred broke the silence, thanking the women for wonderful work. "Alice and her baby are alive, thanks to you. It has been a pleasure working with each of you."

Turning to Annette, Alfred spoke. "As you have just witnessed, nurses and doctors work together, each doing something important for the patient. I want your help inviting college women to become trained nurses. Women such as you."

Once the tea break ended, goodbyes were said, each off to new tasks. Spent, but surprisingly content, Annette left by carriage, returning home.

Returning to her coursework, Annette found focusing challenging. Her experiences with Alfred, Charlotte, and Betty distracted her from her studies. To help bridge her classics coursework to medicine, Annette took from her bookshelf the two volumes of Hippocrates translated by the Scottish physician Francis Adams, published in 1849 and 1886. She was taken with Alfred's reference to "The Oath" on the journey to Alice's home.

While she had been aware of its contents quite generally, she did not know its details. Adams raised some doubt as to its authorship in his 1849 introduction, but the piece seemed to first appear sometime between the second half of the fifth and the first part of the fourth century BC, the Classical Age of Greece. Reading the 1886 annotations, she smiled at the observation by Adams that "there can be no doubt, in short, that the ancients had anticipated all of our modern methods of inducing premature delivery." Alfred would surely disagree. For the sake of Alice and her baby, Alfred must have known, by his "ability and judgement," as the Oath said, that he could do what seemed impossible on a dining room table.

Intrigued, Annette turned to *On Airs, Waters, Places*, with commentary and text in the 1849 volume. Sitting at her desk, Annette became immersed in Hippocrates' associations between seasonal variations, salty versus fresh waters, winds and breezes, sunlight, and disease. Balanced interactions of man and his environment were deemed key to health, Hippocrates' approach to cure emanated from the healing power of nature. Alfred and Hippocrates share the same values, she realized, concepts of medicine that have survived hundreds of years.

On Airs, Waters, Places was short, appearing on pages 190-222. If sufficient copies of Adams could be found, Annette thought the treatise interesting for presentation at her book club. While not all club members would find the reading easy, Annette considered it a stretch worth undertaking. I'll ask Elizabeth her opinion about this idea, she thought, slipping the two volumes in the drawer under her desktop where she kept her most interesting reading.

Her racing thoughts settling, Annette wrote two thank you notes, one to Charlotte Macleod and the other to Alfred Worcester. To Charlotte, Annette asked follow-up questions regarding Alice and her baby boy. Were they healthy? Had Alice recovered from her surgery? Knowing that she did not have enough time to fully appreciate the work of the training school during her first visit, Annette requested to meet with Charlotte again, hoping for details that she might provide her classmates.

Her letter to Alfred was shorter, a simple note of thanks for a most unusual day that heightened her interest in health generally and in nursing more specifically. She asked to join him on another home visit. Perhaps, she wrote, he might be willing to join her classmates for a special session, pending Elizabeth's approval, to talk of health, medicine, and nursing. Ever aware that such unfamiliar topics may seem irrelevant in a classics curriculum, she suggested that writings of Hippocrates might be used as a framework for the session.

Bridges, she knew, would need to be built.

Caroline loved Christmas. It was declared a legal holiday in Massachusetts in 1856, and Caroline knew that this Christmas would be special. She planned to celebrate her son, Philip, and Abigail's anticipated engagement, as well as pursue Alistair Campbell as a possible suitor for Annette. Marguerite, her vivacious middle child, was now succeeding as a special student studying modern languages at the Harvard Annex. And Amos, her hardworking journalist husband, remained at *The Globe*, despite her urging that he return to a more lucrative law career.

At the center of an Episcopalian family, Caroline planned the main holiday celebration on Christmas Eve, with minor festivities enjoyed during the twelve days from December 25th through January 5th, the day before the Epiphany. Swags of garland and holly adorned all fireplaces, door frames, and staircases. A majestically tall Fraser fir tree stood boldly in a corner of the main sitting parlor, decorated with tinsel, pastries in the shape of stars, and popcorn strings looped around the tree. Held in place with an iron tree stand purchased in Pennsylvania years earlier, the tree was secure enough for candied fruit to hang on it. Heralding it a sugar tree, Caroline was proud, claiming that her tree was surely the most beautifully decorated in Cambridge.

Annette and Caroline ventured into Cambridge's main shopping street ten days before the family's Christmas Eve dinner.

"You simply must have a lovely new dress for our dinner, Annie," Caroline said firmly, eyes narrowing. "Alistair will be joining us, and you must look your best." Caroline frowned as Annette arched her eyebrows in response.

Caroline chatted with her favorite dressmaker, whose pin cushion wristband waved perilously in the air, accentuating her words, amid floor-to-ceiling bolts of variously colored fabrics. As the kaleidoscope of color, voices, and movement swirled, Annette perched on a lounge chair at the front of the store, enjoying the warm sun streaming through the glass windows. Reading the December 10th, 1892, issue of *The Women's Journal and Suffrage News* that she had brought with her, she noted that the Graduate Club of the Harvard Annex had recently elected its officers. While she knew these officers, she was not particularly interested in the club itself, given that she had purchased, for two dollars and fifty cents, an annual subscription solely for news on the suffrage movement.

In the past several weeks, Annette felt her life becoming more complex, with thoughts of suffrage (and her aunt Ellen), classics (and her mentor Lizzie), women at Harvard (and President Eliot), and health (Dr. Worcester and Charlotte Macleod) mingling in chaotic ways. Does this happen with age? she wondered. Uncomfortable, yet stimulated by such diverse ideas, Annette decided to embrace the unknown milieu.

"Annie," called Caroline loudly, waking Annette from her reverie, "do pick a dress pattern and color for our dinner at Christmas. I think you would look stunning in a silk magenta dress with a lace bodice. What do you think?" Annette rarely saw her mother so happy as she was today.

"I agree, Mother. A silk magenta evening dress with lace would be lovely."

Annette stood patiently on the dressing room stool as her portly dressmaker pinned her hem, talking all the while with Caroline.

Perhaps, thought Annette, this might be a good time to ask her mother to invite Alfred to her Christmas dinner, as a thank you for his tour of Waltham Hospital.

"That is an excellent idea! We will invite him," said Caroline.

Annette beamed. Promising Caroline that she would return to the store for a fitting in a few days, Annette returned to her lounge chair, combing through the journal for current information on the suffrage movement. Annoyed at finding more advertisements for mattresses, stove polish, food, and medicine than articles on suffrage, she tossed the journal on the small table by the lounge chair, offering free reading for any customer interested in advertisements.

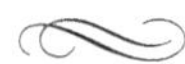

Once home, Annette was thrilled to receive a letter from Charlotte Macleod. Why, she wondered, was she so excited about Charlotte's letter? Sitting at her desk, her most comfortable, secure spot, Annette carefully opened the letter. Two pages long, with delicate Palmer method penmanship, Charlotte's letter was delicious. Almost two months had passed since her visit to Waltham. Perhaps I have been invited to return to the milieu.

Dear Annette,

I was pleased to hear from you. I have so very much to tell you.

Charlotte's voice was warm, welcoming.

Charlotte spoke of Alice and her baby boy, telling Annette that the father never returned, leaving Alice to seek employment and baby care. Charlotte was worried that, if she found neither, Alice would turn to prostitution, taking customers into her apartment. If she became ill, she would require care at an almshouse for the poor. If unable to care for her baby, Alice would then have to place her baby for adoption, consistent with the state's Adoption of Children Act of 1851. Charlotte wrote that many such problems were now plaguing the city, with crowding, industrial accidents, and infectious diseases on the rise.

Annette, have you read Jacob Riis's book, How the Other Half Lives? *What he reports is heartbreakingly true. We see it in our own city.*

Her voice now dark and sad, Charlotte was overwhelmed by the tragedies she had witnessed.

On another note, Annette, you are very welcome to come to the school again. We have much more to talk about. You can bring any classmates with you. I would like to describe our program and clinical rotations of our pupils. We patterned our program on Florence Nightingale's recommendation to follow that of the Metropolitan and National Nursing Association, founded in London in 1875, to provide training for nurses caring for the sick poor. Our program aims to help the people of our community. Our pupil probies first learn in district homes, followed by a year in hospital service, and lastly, a return to home care. I can introduce you to pupils, show you our classroom and pupil dorm rooms, and answer any questions you may have. I'll also update you on what is happening in Massachusetts with registration of nurses, a topic that really rankles Dr. Worcester.

Have a happy Christmas!

Fondly,

Charlotte

Annette folded Charlotte's letter, placing it on her desk to read again after dinner. Alice perhaps in an almshouse and her baby to be placed for adoption, shocking possibilities to Annette. I must ask my father about Jacob Riis's book, she thought. He may even know him personally. From what she experienced with Alice in a tenement, Annette was beginning to understand the interlocking causes and effects of poverty. She was also beginning to appreciate the ways that everyone was, or perhaps should be, connected.

Poverty was only a carriage ride away, and that fact was now in her consciousness.

Wishing to impress Alfred with both her knowledge and initiative and, for her own sake, to learn more about those who were so badly served by society, Annette replied to Charlotte, asking to visit before her mother's Christmas Eve party.

For now, Annette sought her father, hoping to learn more about Jacob Riis and his book. As she entered his library, Annette considered translating pithy sections of Riis's book into both Latin and Greek in her quest to link the ancient world to Cambridge.

"I do know Jacob," said Amos, smiling to his precocious daughter. "He is a very fine writer. Jacob was a police reporter for *The New York Tribune* when I worked for *The Times*. His book, *How the Other Half Lives*, was published in *Scribner's Magazine* at Christmas, 1889. He was one of the first to use flash photography, a new way to clearly illuminate photos in dark settings."

"Some call him a muckraker. I call him a man with a conscience, a true social activist." As he spoke, Amos turned to his floor-to-ceiling bookcases, searching for Riis's name in his carefully organized collection.

"Here it is," Amos said with delight. "Jacob brought much to light through his reporting. His work will help change our cities."

"Why do you ask about Jacob, Annie?" His brilliant daughter generally spoke only of distant worlds, never of Cambridge in the 1890s.

Annette brought Amos to the gazebo in their backyard. It was their safe, quiet space. There, she reviewed her time with Alfred and Charlotte, the patients in the Waltham Hospital, and pregnant Alice in a tenement. She also described Charlotte's letter regarding outcomes for Alice and her baby, her voice less confident than usual.

"Charlotte mentioned Riis's book in her note. She compared his descriptions of New York City tenement life to tenement life in Waltham city. I do want to read Riis's book. It may help me understand the poverty and illness in our state."

"Father," said Annette, continuing, "I find myself as taken with poverty, health, and illness as I am with my study at the Annex. I see amazing similarities between worlds. I admit to being a bit confused, but equally excited to learn of our problems today."

"Journalism is my love, Annie, much to your mother's displeasure. Law might bring more income. Newspaper writing has direct impact. Illuminating issues stimulates change, and generally, change improves lives." Holding his daughter's hand, he encouraged her to remain excited, to change lives for the better. Classics education, he reminded her, would give her historical context against which she might better understand and interpret the world before her.

"Learn everything you can on your next trip to Charlotte Macleod. A new world has now opened for you, Annie."

Visiting Charlotte Macleod a second time, Annette dressed comfortably, in flouncy navy bloomers and a below-the-knee day dress.

After greeting her at the door of Waltham Hospital, Charlotte offered Annette morning tea and biscuits. As before, the air smelled crisp and clean, an odor Annette coined the *hospital aroma*. No dust dared to enter, nor were pets allowed.

Charlotte, thrilled to show Annette pupil rooms, a small library doubling as a sitting parlor, mid-size kitchen serving on occasion as a chemistry laboratory, and one classroom, was almost breathless with pride when they returned to the sitting parlor. Annette held her questions during the tour, jotting them down in a small notepad, a practice she had learned from her father.

"What is your impression of our school, Annette?" Charlotte, eager to hear Annette's impressions, sat at the edge of her large chair, hands clasped tightly on her white apron, eyes fixed on her guest.

Annette, comparing the Annex's Fay House to the Waltham Training School, scrambled for words to compliment her host's building. One had so much of everything, the other so little of the same. Words failing, Annette veered the conversation to the program's coursework.

"You must be very proud of your accomplishments. This is an important school. I would like to learn about your courses, what books you use, your teachers, the rotations pupils take, and jobs open to them after graduation. I hope to describe your program to my classmates when we return to the Annex after the Christmas holiday." Sipping her tea, Annette intended her questions to effectively derail further conversation about the building itself.

Charlotte laughed. "Not books, or at least not so many of them as line the walls of the Annex. In both our school and hospital, the patient always comes first. We do celebrate holidays, but pupils do not have regularly scheduled vacations such as you may have at the Annex. Our patient first principle drives our program. Let me explain more fully." With so much more worldly experience than Annette, it was easy for Charlotte to make her comfortable in a place so far from her own.

Charlotte said that pupils lived at the school and provided patient care. In exchange, physicians such as Dr. Worcester and Dr. Cutler, and others, including herself, provided lectures on select topics. The lectures included all medical specialties, obstetrics, gynecology, medicine, surgery, pediatrics, infectious diseases, and psychiatry. Rotations in the hospital, patient homes, and other settings in the community, such as milk stations, comprised the clinical apprenticeship of pupils.

"Lectures," Charlotte continued, "are scheduled for later afternoons, when physicians have completed medical rounds and home visits. Since lectures are secondary to patient care, a lecture will be rescheduled if there is a patient emergency. This cannot be helped."

As Charlotte discussed the patient first principle, her pride was palpable to Annette. For Charlotte, the end goal was improvement of the patient's health, the pupil a critical link to that accomplishment. At the Annex, Annette thought, I am expected to graduate proficient in classics. There is no goal beyond that.

It might, at first, seem good to be at the center of everything one encountered in the academy, but there were limits. While it is probable, Annette realized, that I may teach after graduation, it is equally possible that I might marry and begin a family. Graduation from the Annex did not imply any larger societal goal. Most simply, society anticipated that she would comport herself as an educated Back Bay woman. She would certainly belong, but she might also equally belong to someone else.

Smiling to mask her confusion, Annette asked to see textbooks pupil nurses read during their studies. Charlotte rose quickly, directing Annette to the two library shelves in the pupils' sitting parlor. The top shelf held several copies of Clara S. Weeks' 1888 *Text-Book of Nursing*, along with copies of Florence Nightingale's 1860 *Notes on Nursing*, Lavinia Dock's 1890 *Text-Book of Materia Medica for Nurses*, and Henry Gray's *Anatomy of the Human Body*. Charlotte added that the Weeks textbook was the primary reference at the school, with the first duty of the nurse defined as absolute obedience to the physician. Annette decided to read that book first. The second shelf held copies of several current issues of medical journals donated by the school's teaching physicians. They were held in specific wooden boxes labeled accordingly. Journals such as *Lancet, Medical Repository*, the weekly *New England Journal of Medicine*, and the weekly *British Medical Journal* overflowed the holding boxes.

"Our journal library is growing rapidly, with physicians contributing past issues of their specialty publications." Charlotte pulled the current monthly issue of the *Index Medicus* off the shelf, a journal she indicated had been applauded as America's greatest contribution to medical knowledge. She noted that the purpose of the *Index*, a monthly compilation of quality scientific journal articles, was to give physicians access to current research and knowledge. The *Index*, begun in 1879 by John S. Billings, director of the Army Surgeon General's library, was, according to Charlotte, a cherished, prized holding.

Annette questioned two other holdings off to the corner of the second shelf, by appearance less read. One was entitled *Plain Directions for the Care of the Sick and Recipes for Sick People*, written in 1875 by Alexander P. Turner and distributed to policy holders of the Mutual Life Insurance Company of New York. Although Charlotte considered it invaluably practical as a patient teaching guide, she offered that it focused more on healthy behaviors than on disease treatment, a focus unattractive to the pupil nurses and not relevant to hospital care. The second holding was a large box labeled "Dr. Worcester's Monthly Nursing Notes." These, according to Charlotte, were Dr. Worcester's lecture notes on obstetrical nursing delivered to pupil nurses at the Lying-In Hospital during his medical school years. At the top of the pile of lecture notes rested a single book of 250 pages entitled *Monthly Nursing*. Charlotte noted that the book was a highly read reference for pupils during their obstetrical rotation.

Annette saw at once why Mutual Life had an interest in wellness. A healthy patient, paying insurance premiums with the devotion that one tithes in church, is pure profit. She wondered if Charlotte knew how men of privilege really worked.

"His lecture notes were published in 1886 by the firm D. W. Mason, after his graduation from Harvard. *Monthly Nursing* is believed to be the first book published in obstetrical nursing. The nurses at the Lying-In Hospital loved him! When he graduated, they hosted a party for him, giving him an umbrella that he continues to use today." Her respect for Alfred impressed Annette, who was beginning to recognize his integral role in Waltham.

She, too, was increasingly impressed by, and interested in, Alfred.

Before Annette left, Charlotte told her that the International Congress of Charities, Correction, and Philanthropy planned several congresses to be held from June 12th through 18th, at the 1893 World's Fair in Chicago. A specific section of the International Congress, according to Charlotte, would be on all matters relating to the hospital care of the sick, the training of nurses, dispensary work, and first aid to the injured. John S. Billing would chair this section. She added that the superintendent of the Johns Hopkins Training School for Nurses, Miss Isabel A. Hampton, would serve as president of the section on training of nurses. Charlotte said that in the upcoming January 28th issue of *The Hospital*, Dr. Billings would encourage any person interested in participating in this section to contact Dr. Henry H. Hurd at the Johns Hopkins Hospital in Baltimore.

"Annette, perhaps you may be interested in attending the section on nurses' training at the International Congress. It will be wonderfully informative. You may learn much about nursing education and registration of nurses, both important topics for our hospital and school. Dr. Worcester plans to attend."

Given the late hour and cloudy afternoon, Annette declined afternoon tea and instead thanked her host and returned home. She was beginning to see the milieu from the inside.

Caroline's house at 1564 Massachusetts Avenue in Cambridge was only a quarter mile from Fay House on Garden Street and even less distance to Harvard. A perfect central location for a prominent family. Ever vigilant about appearances, Caroline, determined to have the most elegantly decorated home for Christmas Eve, looped garland and tinsel around all doors and windows facing the main avenue. Candles adorned each window, with baskets of fresh pine cones and needles strategically placed in the house for maximum aroma. Perhaps, she thought, her home might be pictured on the holiday cover of *Life* magazine, a weekly publication that enjoyed a wide audience. Annette was stationed at the front door to welcome her mother's guests.

The dinner party, according to Annette, included the standard guest list, Ellen and Stubby. Alfred Worcester was the first to arrive, bringing a guest holding a large basket of home-baked cookies, scones, and shortbread.

"My wife, Elizabeth," said Alfred, smiling as he made introductions, "loves to bake at the holidays. And I enjoy her treats, especially with a little Scotch whiskey."

Annette stopped breathing for a moment as the word *wife* broke through and, reaching to take the basket from Alfred, noticed, for the first time, a gold wedding band on his left ring finger.

How had I not noticed this before? she asked herself as a disquieting mixture of embarrassment and jealousy washed over her.

Annette welcomed her guests, closed the door, and followed them into the house, silently taking her place at her mother's dining table. She abandoned her previous plans for intimate conversation with Alfred in favor of polite discussion of Waltham and the sweeping effects of industrialization on that city. After the holiday main meal of baked ham carved on the sideboard; sweet potatoes; candied carrots; and a light salad of romaine lettuce, radishes, and green onions was completed, the dessert was presented in the sitting parlor. The parlor was an unusual place to serve dessert; Caroline wanted her guests to comfortably enjoy the last course while smelling the delicious aroma of her large Christmas tree.

"Elizabeth and Alfred, do you celebrate Christmas?" Caroline sought congenial topics, hoping to engage all guests in pleasant, nonconfrontational conversations.

Elizabeth spoke first.

"My father, Thomas Hill, was a Unitarian minister." In a faltering voice, Elizabeth added that he had been ill for some time and had recently died. She said that he had been Harvard's twentieth president, succeeded by Charles Eliot in 1869. As a Unitarian, she did indeed celebrate Christmas. "It might be said," she added with a laugh, "that we invented the tradition in America."

Annette was taken by Elizabeth's quiet demeanor, her stoic grief, her sense of humor. Clearly, like Annette herself, Elizabeth seemed to have been close to her father. With a small, fragile frame, gray-blue eyes, and long strawberry-blonde hair swept by a bright red ribbon over her left shoulder, Elizabeth impressed Annette. Neither awkward nor boastful, Elizabeth was charming and amiable. Listening to her speak, Annette decided that it would not be worth the effort to dislike her.

By contrast, Alfred's retelling of his religious beliefs was detailed, almost storylike. Fascinated by Alfred's move from Swedenborgianism, or the New Church, to his eventual confirmation as an Episcopalian at Trinity Church in Boston, Amos encouraged Alfred to recall major points of his religious journey. Describing his upbringing in the New Church community, including his early education at the New Church School at Piety Corner, where his father was principal, Alfred noted that his family was firmly rooted in the New Church teachings. His father, Alfred claimed, enjoyed what he termed a state of spiritual receptiveness of the Truth. Alfred recalled, however, growing doubts throughout his years at Harvard about Swedenborg's revelations, particularly his visions with angels and his communications with former inhabitants of the moon.

As Alfred's doubts grew, along with expansion of his scientific knowledge, he became acquainted with Phillip Brooks, an Episcopal clergyman, and eventually joined the Episcopal church, stating that he liked its breadth in including widely differing groups and societies.

"This was a turning point in my life. I celebrated Easter after keeping Lent, and then felt a perfect peace." Once an Episcopalian, Alfred said he ceased obsessing about religion and became engrossed with his family practice in Waltham.

Alfred's youthful involvement with Swedenborgianism intrigued Amos, himself captivated by tales of other worlds. In fact, only one year earlier, Amos published *Reports of a Traveler Returned from The Undiscovered Country*, in which he described experiences as a disembodied entity in an alternate universe.

"Perhaps," Amos mentioned to Alfred, "we can talk again sometime. I would like you to review my recent *Reports* and let me know your thoughts on it." Emanuel Swedenborg claimed to have conversed with former inhabitants of the moon. Similarly, Amos wrote of disembodied experiences in another universe. We may, in fact, have some very interesting conversations over sherry and dessert, thought Amos as he smiled at Alfred and Elizabeth.

I will miss having Alfred to think about in ways I had hoped, Annette thought. A pity I will never see those blue eyes close for sleep.

Walking closer to Caroline's Christmas tree as the conversation waned, Alfred asked if Annette had enjoyed her recent visit with Charlotte Macleod at the Waltham Training School for Nurses.

"I had an absolutely wonderful day with Charlotte," Annette said, happy to see a turn in the conversation. "Charlotte has encouraged me to attend the Chicago World's Fair in a few months, to specifically observe the session on the training of nurses by Isabel Hampton. She said that you may be attending this session also. Is that true?" She did not mention that she had already accepted Alistair's invitation.

As Alfred said that, yes, he planned to attend, Annette observed her mother's scowl.

"Annette," her mother began, "as a student at the Annex, do you need to learn more about nursing? You are quite removed from nurses and hospitals. Remember that nurses are still not held in great regard, some accepting nursing work as punishment for crimes." Caroline could not refrain from commenting, despite Alfred's presence and high praise for nurses. To Caroline, nursing would bring disgrace to the family name.

"Mother, I simply wish to learn more. I had planned to travel to Chicago in summer 1893 to attend the fair. I would enjoy listening to Miss Hampton speak about nursing licensure and registration. Nursing is an interesting, growing field, one offering women other choices in their lives."

For a moment, silence descended until Caroline, always the hostess, broke into a laugh.

"Well," she declared in stage whisper, "at least in a hospital no one will notice your appalling taste in dresses."

Everyone chuckled just enough to let the air back into the room. Annette sat next to Alistair, nudging him with an elbow as she grinned. Ellen smiled at Stubby, quiet after a satisfying meal.

When all the guests had gone, Caroline confronted Amos.

"I hope you forbid Annie from traveling to Chicago. Imagine, wanting to learn about nursing. How disgraceful." Flushed and angry, Caroline paced before the Christmas tree.

"She is a grown woman, my dear, and may do as she wishes."

"And, without a formal engagement to Alistair, Annette simply cannot be in his company for an extended trip. That would not be proper." Caroline was working up steam.

Amos faced Caroline, stopping her in her tracks.

"Caroline, Annette will not marry Alistair."

"And why not?" asked Caroline, feeling suddenly that everyone might know something she did not.

"Alistair's interests lie elsewhere."

"That is absurd, Amos. He adores the company of Annette."

"He does indeed, my dear. But he enjoys the company of men more."

A door had been opened that Caroline did not want to enter. She turned from the tree and headed, alone, into the kitchen.

Realization

"**A**nnette, this is a mistake."

"Mistake? No, this is the first step," countered Annette.

Alfred, flushed, walked from the sitting parlor reserved for the Annex book club meeting to the impressive front doors of Fay House. Leaning on the porch railing outside the main doors, Alfred was disappointed in Annette's classmates' views of Hippocrates's work.

Inside, fifteen of Annette's classmates were on a tea break after a lively discussion of Hippocrates's *On Airs, Waters, Places*, as well as his "Oath." While most had given the two works only a brief cursory read, one had devoured them in the translations by Adams. In the former, she found the links between health and the environment insightful. In the latter, she found the ethical imperative bold.

Millicent Thompson, or Millie to everyone who knew her, was a quiet, reserved student living with her parents in their home on Gerry Street, eight blocks from Fay House. A superior scholar, today she was uncharacteristically enthusiastic about Hippocrates's writing, seeing close parallels between his world and her own. In discussion, she claimed "The Oath" to be a masterpiece of applied moral philosophy.

While one classmate questioned if *masterpiece* was the most appropriate word to characterize "The Oath," all agreed that Adams's translation, given that he was both a physician and a translator, was a worthy endeavor, especially given its wide use in American medicine. There was an animated discussion on ways translation altered meaning. The first half of the meeting ended successfully, with the women trailing off in discussions of etymology and authorship. Alfred and Annette drifted into the parlor.

"Alfred," Annette continued, "the discussion of Hippocrates's work was intended to be an introduction for my colleagues to the Waltham Training School, to the profession of nursing." Contrary to his disappointment, she regarded the discussion as successful, a way to set the context for a later, more focused conversation on hospital care and nursing.

"My classmates and I are classics scholars. We are not at all involved in health. Viewed in this light, I believe they demonstrated amazing interest in Hippocrates's work, at least enough to consider discussing it in terms of applied uses." Annette cautioned Alfred to be realistic, to give her classmates time to understand his work and to explore nursing as a possible profession of interest to college-educated women and those who were college-bound. She reminded him that her own interest in nursing grew over the past few months, particularly given her experiences with him and Charlotte Macleod.

"The book club students are your target audience, your advisors. Your program must attract young women interested in earning a college degree. With their input, your current training school might, perhaps will, become, eventually, a college degree program. These women are not puppets, and you are not their Geppetto." She was piqued. Ushering him to return to the meeting, Annette tapped on Elizabeth Agassiz's office door to inform her that Alfred's portion of the meeting was about to start. Annette and Alfred returned to the club room, with Elizabeth taking the lead.

Tea completed, the students returned to their comfortable reading chairs, awaiting Alfred's overview of the Waltham Hospital and Training School for Nurses. Elizabeth, clearly leading activities in the room, was seated in a large French wing armchair, providing an elegant atmosphere to the club meeting. Smiling, she told her audience that Alfred was a friend to the Annex and an alumnus of Harvard's Medical School.

"President Charles Eliot, Alfred Worcester, and I have met on several occasions, frequently exploring educational opportunities for women. I am fully versed in Dr. Worcester's work at Waltham. He is here today to introduce you to the field of nursing and to seek your advice on nursing education as a possible professional path to women like yourselves at the Annex and our seven sister colleges." Gesturing to Alfred, Elizabeth sat back in her armchair, pencil and small silver and bone notepad, with attached loop for waistband carrying, in her hands.

Alfred awkwardly rose from his armchair, thanking Elizabeth and the students for the luxury of their time. With piercing slate-blue eyes, dark-brown hair parted in the center and curling over ears and nape of neck, Alfred, in his dark-charcoal brushed cotton frock coat, vest, broad black tie and crisp white shirt, was the epitome of style and sophistication. His presence captivated the room. Sensing this, Alfred's confidence blossomed, and he warmed easily to an overview of both hospital and school. Opening with reference to

Charles Dudley Warner and Mark Twain's novel *The Gilded Age: A Tale of Today*, he quickly sequenced rapid industrialization, urbanization, materialistic excess countered by poverty, and, ultimately, the need for organized health care and hospitals.

Alfred held their attention.

"Health care has historically been a function of families," he said. "Night watchers and friendly visitors helped families care for sick relatives. Our needs now overwhelm families." Physicians, he described, would previously secure services of private-duty nurses listed on registries. These nurses, some trained and some not formally trained, lived with families and managed the ill patient, in addition to helping with light domestic duties. As contagious diseases, including tuberculosis, diphtheria, typhoid fever, and scarlet fever, spread rapidly in crowded cities and tenements, hospitals were established to safely treat severely ill patients, including those injured in industrial accidents.

"Ill patients," Alfred emphasized, "are cared for by pupil nurses in hospitals. Using tools from scientific discoveries and sanitary science, pupil nurses apprentice in hospital wards, caring for patients under the tutelage of physicians." Patients improve, he proposed, only if well-trained pupil nurses provide effective care. Alfred noted that most pupil nurses became employed as private-duty nurses once they completed their program. Some, he added, did enter public health nursing, given that state departments of health were becoming established, with local programs requiring nursing for well-care efforts, vaccination programs, and childcare stations. Hospital care was delivered by pupil nurses, operating under the patient first motto. Physicians and pupil nurses cared for patients first, with teaching of pupils a secondary activity as time permitted.

His audience listening intently, Alfred ventured to describe the nursing curriculum and lifestyle. Admission requirements for most training schools, he mentioned briefly, included a minimum age of twenty-one, with the oldest no more than thirty-five; evidence of a common school education; good health; and strong common sense. Most schools also required that pupils be unmarried and without children. The Waltham School's curriculum included one year of probationary work, elementary sciences, and class lectures. Throughout the program, pupils learned hospital nursing as well as district nursing and home care. Rotations in baby care and other specialties were also included, as was industrial nursing at local factories.

"The purpose of our school is purely educational. It is independent of any hospital's needs or advantages. The year of hospital nursing is to teach illness nursing, and thus, to save students from mechanical hospitalism."

"Hospitals," Alfred stressed, "are not educational institutions."

Taking a deep breath, Alfred finished his overview. Turning to Annette, he asked her to describe her recent visit to the hospital and school, as well as her home visit to Alice, his pregnant patient living in a Waltham tenement. Annette, pleased to describe her experiences, found herself pacing as she excitedly relayed events of her tours.

"My experiences transported me from ancient Greece and Rome to Waltham, Cambridge, Boston."

"I feel alive."

As she spoke, Annette's long hair had loosened from her ribbon. Quietly pulling her hair into place, she took her seat between Elizabeth and Alfred.

"Well," said Elizabeth, "comments, questions, anyone?" Scanning the room, Elizabeth sensed a mix of excitement and discomfort. What are we to do with this information? she imagined them thinking, with emotions ranging from fascination to annoyance. Indeed, she noted, several students were sitting upright, almost on the edge of their chairs, attracted to the allure of nursing, wanting more stories. A few, in contrast, seemed displeased, gathering their belongings as if wanting to leave as soon as possible.

Millie, who thrived on details, began the conversation.

"I have enjoyed learning about what nurses do, how they function in different places, how they work in teams with physicians and others. But I simply can't envision where they live, what their coursework involves, how they rotate from hospital work to patient homes, what the relationship is between the hospital and the school." A believer, Millie sought clarification. She always wanted answers to her reasonable questions.

Answers would be complex, thought Annette. She found herself frequently returning to her times with Alfred, Charlotte, and Betty during her brief tours in Waltham. Nursing was complicated work, involving intimate relationships with patients and their families. Nurses, it seemed to Annette, managed health, while physicians managed disease. Something, however, seemed absent, even inappropriate, in the education of nurses.

Who took the place of these women? To be both pupil and functioning nurse at the same time was indefensible, a situation too untenable to be termed education. The hours were extreme, the living arrangements bordered on servitude, the patient first principle when held as a creed diminished learning, and the apprenticeship approach lacked rigor. The relationship between hospitals and training schools was surely an inappropriate one, she reasoned, even in the gilded age of capitalism as income flowed to hospitals for the work conducted by pupil nurses. The formal rules of obedience to the physician and absolute adherence to hospital practices, both professed by Clara Weeks in her nursing textbook, contrasted sharply with intellectual inquiry, a mark of true education. Would Charles Eliot deem nursing training schools as education at its best?

Gazing quickly at Alfred, Annette realized that he did not have answers for Millie. Nor did she.

"Millie, your questions are important and practical. For today, we will address your questions indirectly, by first considering nursing as a university offering." To secure her classmates' continued interest, Annette decided to shift the conversation quickly, from hospitals to the Annex. "Lizzie, can nursing be offered at the Annex, similarly to the classics? At Harvard, both dentistry and medicine are degree programs. How do dental and medical students receive their training with patients?"

Annette's questions flabbergasted Elizabeth. Caught without predetermined responses, Elizabeth answered frankly.

"Yes, Annette, the Annex may be able to offer nursing as a program, as Harvard offers both medicine and dentistry. Nursing is surely the third leg of the proverbial three-legged health stool." Seeming lost in thought, eyes musing on the notepad in her hand, Elizabeth abruptly stood up. Smoothing her full-length simple deep-blue skirt with blouse sleeves puffed out broadly in her upper arm, Elizabeth slowly scanned each student present.

"To offer nursing," Elizabeth said, "much preliminary work would need to be undertaken." Expanding, Elizabeth gestured in the air with her pencil, detailing steps to be taken for nursing to be offered at the Annex. Settling her eyes on Alfred, Elizabeth reminded the group that the Annex must be authorized to award degrees, otherwise training would remain the rule of the day.

Elizabeth allowed a brief side conversation on differences between education and training prior to outlining other tasks to be accomplished. Most critically, she noted, the roles of nurses in various settings must be understood and recognized, along with the relationships between and among nurses, physicians, dentists, and others who cared for families. If such roles were understood, then other factors could be explored in detail, including admissions criteria, the curriculum, faculty requirements, faculty availability, library resources, practical experiences, contracts with patient settings, tuition and other costs, and recruitment efforts. Relationships with hospitals, home care registries, district nursing associations, industrial sites, and other sites for rotational experiences would have to be solidified. Certainly, she stressed, work would need to be undertaken. In concluding, she allowed for a bright future.

"Yes, it is possible to offer nursing at the Annex."

Millie was first on the uptake. "If nursing was an Annex program, then perhaps students might enroll," she proposed. Students began talking at once, citing interest in nursing if offered by the Annex in much the same manner that medicine and dentistry were offered by Harvard. "Women today want to be educated, to vote, to have their voices heard," Millie said, reflecting her classmates' thoughts, or at least, she thought wily, those who believed education as something other than a finishing school.

Book club members thanked Alfred, Elizabeth, and Annette for a lively meeting. The students gave their polite applause. As they began to leave, Alfred overheard one say to another that the old fellow was in the wrong place to recruit servants.

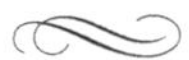

In his 17 Quincy Street home in Cambridge, reserved to house Harvard presidents, Charles Eliot was ordinarily relaxed, comfortably in control. The house had been his home since becoming president in 1869, with alterations and enlargement undertaken at the request of his second wife, Grace Hopkinson, in 1877. Much of the furniture was his mother's, furniture that had survived his father's bankruptcy in the panic of 1857 and now provided him a sense of private contentment in his otherwise highly public life. Keenly aware that his official station gave him a curious power of influence, he recognized that such power should be wielded for ethically informed progress. As he learned from his fictional hero Rollo in the children's series *Rollo Books* by Jacob Abbott, moral conduct is a primary characteristic of a Christian.

Today, however, Charles was not comfortable in his home.

Pacing slowly in front of the fireplace in his sitting parlor, Charles looked at his hands, fingers laced in a tight grip with only an occasional glance at his pocket watch. While he had requested that his sister, Catherine Storer, serve as his hostess for the present meeting given that his wife, Grace, was out of town visiting family, he requested that Catherine return home once he understood the true purpose of the visit. Upon entering the sitting parlor, Elizabeth Agassiz said that she, Alfred Worcester, and Annette Fiske had a proposal for women's education, specifically, nursing education, to review with him. Realizing that the visit would be neither social nor pleasant, Charles, dismissing social etiquette, asked the kitchen maid to bring only tea for his guests. He wanted to move this meeting out of his schedule and those who requested it out of his home.

Did they not understand the sheer complexity of the topic? he wondered. Did they recognize the discord, the cacophony of noise stimulated by the seemingly simple phrase *women's education*? As he took his seat in the large armchair by the fireplace, Charles smiled, thinking of his statement to his friend Daniel C. Gilman, first president of Johns Hopkins University, that the customs of faculty are those of porcupines on the defensive. We may be dealing with porcupines soon, he thought.

While Elizabeth introduced nursing education for women as the main reason for their visit, Charles understood the full context. Women's college education, nursing schools, hospitals, physicians, health insurance companies, politics, and more. The myriad of factors that must invariably be acknowledged on this topic required one thing that might be insufficient: time. Transforming the professional standards of the medical school had taken more than two years, with changes to examinations, structured clinical rotations, abandonment of the self-selected apprenticeship model, and financial restructuring. By 1871, the school catalogue indicated that the plan of study had changed, an understatement announcing a revolution in medical school education.

As Elizabeth, Alfred, and Annette balanced teacups on their laps, Charles asked, "What shall we turn to first in your plan to open up all fronts at once?"

Clearing her throat amidst the chilliness in the room, Elizabeth began. "Charles, it is time to begin. However well, or poorly, we must begin," Elizabeth said calmly.

She had known Charles since her late husband Louis had been appointed professor at Harvard in 1859. Prior to his installation as Harvard's president in 1869, Charles had been appointed to the chemistry laboratory of Harvard's Lawrence Scientific School in

1860, where Louis had previously served as its head. Elizabeth recalled, smiling only to herself, that Charles angrily resigned from his Harvard position in 1863 when he was not selected for the Rumford Professorship of Chemistry, a position he coveted, viewing himself as the most intellectually capable candidate for the position. Saying at the time that he had been "shamefully wronged by the corporation of Harvard," Charles also refused a professorship in chemistry at the Lawrence Scientific School, offered by Harvard's president Thomas Hill, Alfred Worcester's father-in-law.

Charles, beyond competitive, must be first in everything. Elizabeth knew this, and now she planned to use this knowledge to her benefit.

She began by describing that which Charles knew: There were six private colleges for women in Massachusetts, New York, and Pennsylvania, all claiming to be comparable to prestigious male institutions. These colleges, she stressed, had offered women's education before Harvard, with Mount Holyoke College established first, in 1837. Alfred added that hospitals were being built rapidly, with training schools of nursing established to provide around-the-clock care. He saw a connection.

"Charles, I was among the first classes to graduate from Harvard's restructured medical school in 1883." Alfred affirmed that he was prepared to practice as a physician, given Harvard's organized program, well-planned rotations, and excellent faculty. "But physicians," he confessed, "cannot stay the course of health care alone."

Alfred gave a brief summary description of the role of nurses in health care. They provide direct patient care, as well as education to families for continued good health. They require education, not training. Their first duty is to the patient, not obedience to the physician. Physicians and nurses practice as teams. A nurse's place is at the bedside, in the home, and in public service. Their education must parallel the structure of medical education, rather than monastic servitude. Training solely in hospitals serves only the hospital, as they recover patient revenue and maintain a workforce of unpaid pupil nurses. Nursing students, like medical students, can pay tuition for their education.

Unconsciously, Alfred had stood up, pacing in front of the fireplace, hands gesturing for emphasis. Flushed, he settled himself back in his armchair. Charles found his ways winning.

"Annette, what are your thoughts?" Charles had noted that Annette had withdrawn her chair slightly behind Alfred's and Elizabeth's chairs, as if to signal her lesser position in the group.

"You are a possible target of this conversation. What do you think of a college degree in nursing?"

As was her custom, Annette answered frankly.

"My classmate Millie said it succinctly. If nurses are critical to health, then they require formal college education." She briefly described her experiences in Waltham as confirmation of Millie's conclusion.

Annette continued. "If Harvard is to offer college education to prepare nurses, then it must first offer college education to women." Glancing at Elizabeth, Annette gestured for her to continue this thread in the conversation.

"When will the Annex be empowered to grant degrees, Charles? What must we do to make this happen?"

He realized that this agenda item was not going to go away. He recalled, with a wince, his own claim in his inaugural speech twenty-three years ago that the world knew next to nothing about the natural mental capacities of the female sex. He knew that he was wrong in believing that generations of civil freedom and social equality were needed to obtain the data necessary for an adequate discussion of women's natural tendencies, tastes, and capabilities. But now, he was sure that the best people to lead the campaign were balancing teacups in his parlor.

"Elizabeth," he conceded, "it is time for us to bring together members of the Society for the Collegiate Instruction of Women and fellows of Harvard College to discuss the status of women at the Annex." Charles reviewed the next steps to be undertaken if the Society members and the Harvard fellows agreed to pursue education for women. Noting that the Annex had been moving in the direction of degree-granting since 1879, he indicated that the next logical step would be to apply to the commonwealth for the Harvard Annex to award degrees.

As he spoke, Charles had moved to the front window. "We are, in fact, late in applying, given that six other institutions have moved forward ahead of us. Nevertheless, we are ready now. Our Harvard faculty have accepted female students at the Annex, and they have proven stellar in their academic performance."

Charles and Elizabeth agreed that two steps were needed. The Annex must be granted authority to award degrees, and Harvard must establish a school of nursing along the lines of the medical and dental schools. Neither were easy tasks, but they were forward-thinking and necessary. Charles knew that time would be an enemy, but he also knew that those leading the charge were formidable. It was now winter, 1893. Perhaps the Annex would be authorized to award academic degrees in 1894, and, with aggressive planning, a Harvard school of nursing may be established by the turn of the century.

"Harvard was not the first university to admit women, but it will be the first to establish a school of nursing," Charles proclaimed.

As Annette and Alfred listened, Charles and Elizabeth confirmed dates for meetings between the Society and the Harvard fellows, with a cursory outline of steps to be taken.

"We are the core planning team," said Charles. "We'll meet every Monday morning at 7 am in my office to make sure we stay on course and execute next steps efficiently. There are three foci to explore in detail. Elizabeth and I will manage degree-granting authorization for the Annex, and Alfred and Annette will develop a nursing curriculum for a Harvard school of nursing. Manage these on your own. Together, we will determine political strategies for the school's establishment. Come prepared with possible actions to achieve our goals. Annette, bring your classmate Millie, if you wish. She seems useful."

"Charles," Alfred added, "I have been told by Charlotte Macleod, the Waltham Training School nursing superintendent, that nurse leaders believe that training must be conducted in hospitals, not in colleges. We should anticipate resistance."

"Yes, Alfred," Charles responded slowly, cautiously, "we will surely have resistance. Hospital administrators, physicians, medical faculty, nurse administrators, and others with stakes in the status quo will fight us. But we will prevail, as our cause is just."

By the time they left the room, Charles had incorporated the campaign into his schedule. He moved to other business.

Waiting in the outer parlor of Fay House in late January for Alfred to join them, Annette and Millie huddled close to the fire as brutally cold air and freezing hail bombarded the wood-framed structure, creating howling winds, threatening windows.

As they waited, both reviewed Francis Greenleaf Allinson's 1889 *Greek Prose Composition*, a suggested new book highly recommended by their Harvard faculty. Both Annette and Millie adored their classics curriculum, yet health, generally, and nursing, specifically, were fast competing for time and attention. The classics remained a calming, pleasant, private world, distinct from Eliot's fast-paced, urgent, group meetings.

"So sorry for my lateness." The cold from the opened door startled both women.

Alfred, drenched, removed his black Wellington boots, leaving them on the porch. Annette sensed that his usual buoyant confidence was lagging. Yet he could not help but smile at the two young women standing before him. Annette's chestnut-brown hair was dotted with snow. She stood imperially straight and towered over Millie, whose woolen beret, pulled forward with her dark-chocolate hair tucked under, made her look like a newsboy.

"Are you well?" Annette asked hesitatingly, hoping that she was not overstepping.

"I am well enough," he replied. "Perhaps later, after our planning discussion, may I stay for a brief time so we may talk?" Annette quickly agreed, quite curious as to possible topics for their chat.

Attention shifted to their task of designing the curriculum for the planned Harvard School of Nursing. They had decided that Saturday mornings suited their schedules best, given that all three already had busy weekday agendas. Charles and Elizabeth, focusing efforts on the Annex's degree-granting status, would work on their agenda according to their own schedules.

Alfred, Annette, and Millie sat in the kitchen, a spacious room with large windows; a table with capacity for ten; and pots, pans, and utensils swaying from the ceiling on large hooks close to the ovens. Clean white aprons hung from hooks behind the entrance door. An inviting aroma permeated this room, so central to the lives of those who lived and worked in the house. In one corner, a floor-to-ceiling spice rack decorated the room, with multiple jars of spices, many of which neither Annette nor Millie had heard of previously. Freshly baked breads, scones, and rolls were laid out on another corner table, with towels covering them to retain freshness. The room was a perfect place to conjure a future. Given the early hour of their Saturday sessions, Annette thought the room perfect for their meetings.

"I am here, Alfred, and I wish to participate, but I don't know nursing. My brief visits to Waltham with you and Charlotte Macleod only introduced me to the subject, one very far from my scope of knowledge."

Annette leaned across the large kitchen table, looking directly at Alfred. "How can I help when I am so ignorant?"

"Uninformed, true, but not ignorant," quipped Alfred. He reassured her that another visit with Charlotte would help fill gaps and address outstanding questions that either she or Millie might have, particularly concerning patient rotations, classroom learning, required textbooks, and pupil lifestyle.

"We will learn as we go."

Charlotte, Alfred expanded, had begun to inform him on the politics of nursing. He learned that Isabel Hampton was a respected nursing leader, appointed in 1889 as the superintendent of the training school for nurses at Johns Hopkins Hospital. Isabel, a

Canadian teacher in her youth, graduated from New York City's Bellevue Hospital Training School for Nurses ten years earlier.

"Just this year," he continued, "Isabel Hampton's textbook, *Nursing: Its Principles and Practice, for Hospital and Private Use*, was published by W. B. Saunders, a very reputable firm in Philadelphia." Alfred claimed that it was an amazing book, one useful for medical students for foundational study. He added that William Osler, a physician who had chaired the committee hiring Isabel at Johns Hopkins, thought she was brilliant, describing her as "an animated Greek statue."

Alfred reminded Annette that Isabel would be chairing the new subsection on nursing within Section III of the International Congress of Charities, Correction and Philanthropy, to be held in Chicago from June 12th through the 18th later that year. Section III, named *Hospital Care of the Sick, Training of Nurses, Dispensary Work, and First Aid to the Injured*, would surely include, according to Alfred, the essentials of a nursing curriculum.

"I will need more than only these essentials," Annette said, smiling broadly. "I want to read nursing textbooks, review current program structures, admission criteria, and direct patient training. My experiences thus far point to a lackluster apprenticeship approach and classroom teaching given only in the absence of patient care." While she had browsed through the few books in the Waltham nursing school library, Annette had not thoroughly read them, nor had she been able to construct a clear picture of a nurse's practice, other than that of a mere assistant to a physician.

Annette peppered Alfred with questions. Who teaches nursing pupils? Are physicians simply training their assistants to alleviate their patient burden? Is the hospital replacing the university as the place of learning?

"If we are to be successful, Alfred, nurse education must occur within a university, not a hospital. Bedside experiences can be structured in *any environment* where people live or work. A school may affiliate with various hospitals, including specialties such as women and children, babies, mental care, and others. Can we not mirror Harvard's medical school structure, rather than emulate a structure demanding obedience, the first principle for Clara Weeks?"

Alfred was silent.

He agreed that nursing education deserved a university setting, with award of degrees at graduation. Hospitals, Alfred believed, were simply sites for patient experiences, as were public health departments, city dispensaries, and others. She was right, of course, he thought. But we are at the very ground level. First, college education for women, and second, academic degrees to practice nursing. The crush of these goals was both thrilling and frightening.

Alfred smiled at Annette, thinking that, together, they were smarter than most people in any room.

"Annette, perhaps the emulation you suggest might begin by parsing roles. While hospitals are a striking instance of our advancing civilization, built to improve care and to manage infection, their function is to cater to illness. The role of the physician involves diagnostics and treatment of illness. As with their roles, their location is often fixed. Nurses have a different, broader, fluid role in maintaining, restoring, and advocating health for both individuals and the public. Nurses are not necessarily bound to place. Their location is relative."

Feeling radical and brave, Annette condensed Alfred's thoughts to a four-word mantra: physician—illness, nurse—health. The more she considered the role of nursing, the more she realized that education, suffrage, employment, and contribution must become available to women. She resolved to join her Aunt Ellen at the upcoming regional meeting of the General Federation of Women's Clubs in Boston. Our goals for the Annex and nursing are intertwined with those of the Federation, she realized, particularly suffrage and contribution.

Turning to the matter at hand, Annette asked Millie if she would travel with Alfred and her to the Chicago World's Fair in June to attend the first Nurses' Congress offered under Isabel Hampton's leadership. Since the Congress would be held during the Annex's summer break, Millie responded enthusiastically, offering any additional support she could provide in the meantime. Annette then told Millie about Alistair and, to the surprise of Alfred, that he would also be travelling with them.

I might, Annette thought with a smile, be a thing with feathers after all.

Until she was invited to Charles's planning team, Millie's involvement in a world beyond the ancients occurred through the lens of *Life*, a magazine that had begun publishing in 1883, when she was a child. Especially enjoying the illustrations, Millie still awaited the arrival of the weekly magazine, a radical diversion from her beloved classics. While not a Gibson Girl herself, Millie admired what the personification intended to represent—the new, educated, independent woman of the late nineteenth century.

Millie knew she was different from Annette, that she brought a unique perspective to the group—a practical view of life, with an understanding of diverse people and classes, and daily lives quite dissimilar to many Back Bay residents. An only child of working parents committed to their daughter's education, Millie made her own bed, washed her dishes, and helped with household chores.

Annette had a broad big-picture view of Charles's two goals.

Millie, conversely, viewed the goals at street level.

Together, they were complementary.

Millie left Fay House first, and Annette and Alfred remained at the kitchen table sipping second cups of tea. Alfred said that he was pleased that Annette had begun reading the textbook by Weeks and that she should continue on to those by Hampton and Dock, as well as the Nightingale classic.

"I will also provide the three-year nursing program plan from the Waltham School, as well as that of the New England Hospital for Women and Children Training School for Nurses, founded in 1872." The New England school, Alfred recalled, was the first training school for nurses in America, modeled after Nightingale's principles of sanitation, hygiene, nutrition, and ventilation. In his work at the Lying-In Hospital in Boston, Alfred was proud to recount his interactions with Linda Richards, the first trained American nurse who had graduated from the New England Hospital for Women and Children Training School for Nurses. After graduating in 1873, Richards became a nursing superintendent at Boston City Hospital, sometimes interacting with Alfred as a consulting obstetrician.

Speaking of Linda Richards awoke keen memories of her poor writing ability, attributed by Alfred to her lack of early education. Asked by her to edit her writing, Alfred complied, becoming aware over time that, as he told Annette, her literacy was wanting.

"Vivid descriptions," he noted, "were very short of punctuation and capitals. Frankly, her writing embarrassed me."

He felt that basic literacy, the ability to write without error and to read fluently, must be a basic requirement for nurses. Now in a reminiscent mood, Alfred described the nurses training program he had initiated at the Lying-In Hospital, including his lectures on obstetrical care, which were later published as *Monthly Nursing*.

"I based my teaching on Nightingale's principles," he said proudly, "sanitary science and bacteriology being most important. I will give you a copy of my book as well."

Prior to the next meeting at Charles Eliot's house, Annette planned to review the nursing textbooks and digest the current structures of the Waltham and New England hospital training programs.

Business complete, Annette turned to Alfred.

"Do you still wish to talk, Alfred?"

"I know that it is quite cold today, but can we take a short walk?" Alfred suddenly seemed nervous, jittery, in the kitchen. Since pacing helped him grapple with anxiety, Annette put on her dark-brown great coat, red and orange muffler, and gloves, saying that she would like a brisk walk.

"Elizabeth had her sixth miscarriage several days ago."

Stopping abruptly to look at her, Alfred told Annette that he and Elizabeth, now married seven years, wanted a family, with a large spacious home and several children. But that dream was not to be. Elizabeth, he said, could become pregnant, but was unable to carry the pregnancy to full term, usually miscarrying between three and four months. Given his medical school practice in the Lying-In Hospital, Alfred had many experiences with birth, maternal morbidity, and stillbirth, but never miscarriage, or spontaneous abortion. He was at a loss. As well, age was not on their side. She was now thirty-eight years old and he thirty-nine. He would remain a doctor, possibly with an appointment to Harvard's medical school in time. She would continue to tutor children in language and piano. Yet their lives, he thought, might never be full, might remain unfinished.

"I only now understand that Elizabeth believes that her baby died within her. She is beyond sorrow. Devastated. She tells me that she has failed me."

Alfred continued, describing Elizabeth's pain, and his.

"I have my work and will survive this loss, but I fear that Elizabeth's dreams for our future are crushed. She is deeply saddened."

Alfred described Elizabeth's desire for children, family dinners, cheerful holidays, partnership with her husband, music, and community service. She desperately wanted what her five siblings had been given. Wondering out loud, he mused that, perhaps, Elizabeth would feel joy in helping sick children, serving as a volunteer at the Baby Hospital.

"Annette, my family has deep roots in Massachusetts. I am the ninth generation of the Worcester family in America. My earliest ancestor, Reverend William Worcester, relocated to Boston from England in 1639 for religious freedom. While I am one of eight children, I know now that my own line ends with me. It will be left to my remaining brothers to carry on the name, to continue the Worcester legacy."

"What shall be my legacy?" Alfred said quietly as he continued walking. "How will Elizabeth and I continue, both feeling such overwhelming loss? Loss of our dream of family, of legacy." Then he fell silent. Annette thought of the lines from Christina Rossetti's poem:

In the bleak mid-winter
Frosty wind made moan,
Earth stood hard as iron,
Water like a stone.
Snow had fallen, snow on snow,
Snow on snow,
In the bleak mid-winter
Long ago.

Annette listened, understanding that her presence was all she could offer at this moment. All she could do was stand beside him. Like Elizabeth, she viewed miscarriage as death. And, given that they would cease efforts at childbearing, she realized they were also burying their dream of family.

After walking in silence, she spoke.

"Alfred, may I offer a thought?"

"I hope you can, Annette," said Alfred in a quiet, monotone voice.

"Perhaps it will be that your legacy shall be the establishment of a Harvard school of nursing. At Harvard, nurses will be educated, not trained. Patients, families, the public will receive good care, focused on health, not disease management. Charles Eliot cannot do this alone. You must be the architect."

Alfred looked up, wondering how Annette, a young, bookish woman, could be so wise.

"You have given me a glimmer of hope. If I can continue, if my sadness can lift, then I know I can help Elizabeth find peace."

Together, they imagined a life for Elizabeth without children, from teaching languages to performing publicly. Annette spoke of her sister, also a lover of language and music. Perhaps, she suggested, we may soon introduce them, watching what may become of their friendship.

Annette and Alfred found themselves back at Fay House. Alfred turned to his carriage and went home to Elizabeth in a house too large for them.

Once home, Annette returned to her desk. It was already dusky outside, with a gentle, deepening glow of orange-red sky rising in the west.

Nursing, Alfred, Charles, and Harvard had begun to draw her close, she realized, with her other responsibilities withdrawing in the wake of these powerful forces. Committed to completing both her current baccalaureate and future master's degree in the classics, Annette struck a bargain with herself. To continue working with these men, she would sacrifice her library time for reading not directly related to her coursework. This, she thought, was not a difficult bargain, though she would miss modern poetry.

She drifted downstairs to the kitchen.

Her mother, characteristically, was there.

"Annie, you are so busy these days,"

Annette, finding most female conversation as banal and superficial, avoided chats with her mother. Turning to the topic of Annette's involvement with Alfred and nursing, Caroline hinted at possible impropriety, given that he was married.

"I wonder, are you more interested in nursing or Alfred?"

With a slight flush warming her cheeks, Annette was surprised at her mother's ability to see such things. She quickly turned the conversation toward Eliot's planning team, its goals, endorsed also by Elizabeth Agassiz. Here was safe conversation.

"This will inevitably become a political effort," said Caroline. Her mother continued to amaze.

"You may wish to speak with both your father for his legal insights and Alistair for his knowledge of local politicians. Charles has friends in high places, but you may also need friends at ground level. These may be people that Amos and Alistair know."

"Annette," Caroline said softly, touching Annette's hand, "you deserve an education. And, while I am not a suffragist, I do understand your cause. I am not quite the mindless hostess you take me to be. "

Then, as if removing herself from her daughter's confidence, she continued. "Your father has told me that you will not marry Alistair, but I am nevertheless exploring other possible suitors for you to consider."

Caroline returned to family business. Ellen had left a message for Annette. The next meeting of the Boston group of the General Federation of Women's Clubs would be held at Ellen's house in a few days.

"Ellen hopes that you will attend the next meeting." Frowning, Caroline said that the main item on the agenda was women's suffrage, as well as something about charities.

"Did Ellen leave any other information, Mother?"

"She mentioned two names, Lillian Wald and Lavinia Dock. Both are social activists and suffragists. And both are nurses. Apparently, these things run together now."

Struggling to refrain from smiling, Annette said that she had heard these names previously and would be very pleased to hear them present.

After a pause, Caroline told Annette that Ellen looked very tired. "You may wish to discourage her from smoking," said Caroline, with an arched eyebrow looking at her daughter. Annette had no idea that her mother knew of Ellen's smoking. Does she know that I smoke also? Perhaps, she thought, mother knows more than she lets on.

Ellen's home in Cambridge, on the corner of Beacon and Kirkland Streets, was a short five-to-ten-minute walk to Harvard Yard. The house itself, with wide wooden planks painted light yellow, had two stories, six bedrooms, two parlors each with fireplaces, several water closets, two storage rooms, and a massive kitchen with attached dining room. It was well lit, with windows in every room covered only by decorative valence curtains. The dining room, with a half-circular wall bordering a yard Ellen called their playground, could accommodate twelve guests at a massive, sprawling oak table. Stubby relished the proximity of their home to his office, a short journey he would take either by walking or by bicycle, and he loved their garden. For Ellen, the house was large enough for her four children, all born within a six-year span. Now, almost three decades later, with children grown and living independent lives, the house was bright but empty, requiring significant maintenance. Stubby's books, ballads, and personal papers had gradually encroached into several rooms, turning children's rooms into libraries.

While Ellen wanted a smaller home, she knew that Stubby was as married to their house as he was to her. Resigned, Ellen made the most of her large house, employing it for women's meetings, Annex student gatherings, suffrage events, and other community functions. While her Sedgwick inheritance legacy income was dwindling, Stubby's academic salary would remain adequate to cover costs, as long as they remained frugal.

Today, Ellen was tired, with an indolent, annoying dry cough that had plagued her for the past few weeks, a malady she treated with hot tea, honey, and whiskey. While the tea, occasionally with whiskey, relaxed and warmed her, it did nothing for the cough and lethargy. Still, today's meeting, she thought, promised to be invigorating.

Claire Williams had previously provided club members with brief biographies of the two guests for the late winter 1893 meeting. Lillian Wald, a nurse, graduated from the New York Hospital Training School for Nurses in 1891. Prior to the club meeting, Wald had begun a visiting nurse service for immigrant residents, many of whom were Russian Jews, in New York City's Lower East Side. Relocating to a simple tenement apartment in the area to be closer to her patients, Wald began what she coined "public health nursing," the integration of nursing care within whole communities. Her charitable work, originally financed by her family, was becoming recognized by others, including philanthropists.

Similarly, Lavinia Dock, an 1886 graduate of New York City's Bellevue Hospital Training School for Nurses, was an outspoken social activist, nurse, and suffragist. A writer, Dock had published a pharmacologic textbook, financed by her father, for nurses. Drawn to the poor, Dock embraced public health, acknowledging the relationship between health, environment, and lifestyle.

Ellen imagined that her niece would find both Wald and Dock intriguing, especially given recent conversations she had reported about health care and nursing with Charles, Alfred, and Elizabeth. From her own perspective, Ellen looked forward to hearing Dock speak on women's rights and suffrage, topics important to her. She hoped her own energy would survive the meeting.

Annette was the first to arrive, with Millie joining them shortly thereafter.

"Smoke?" asked Ellen.

The three women retreated to folding lounge chairs with footrests in Ellen's backyard, inhaling deeply on their hand-rolled cigarettes, their torches of freedom, before other members arrived. Still new to cigarette smoking, Millie coughed a little. They all chuckled. For a moment, they were alone, an island in the stream.

Once club members arrived, settling in armchairs and enjoying tea and scones served by the kitchen maid, Ellen read Claire Williams's report from the previous meeting in fall, 1892. Annette was disappointed to learn that New Jersey had not yet passed a law allowing women admission to the bar. Mary Philbrook continued her battle, with lawyers Lelia Robinson and Anna Christy Fall as advisors. Annette was learning, however, that such battles take time, and persistence.

As Ellen directed members' attention to new items on the agenda, Lillian Wald and Lavinia Dock were directed to the meeting parlor. An unusual pair, Lavinia and Lillian, while both nurses, appeared radically unlike.

Despite her affluent background, Lillian, twenty-six years old, lived by choice in a New York tenement on Jefferson Street with her nursing colleague Mary Brewster. With average height, light-brown hair swept into a haphazard bun on top of her head, rather drab attire, and a well-padded waistline, Lillian presented as a soldier, ready and willing to serve.

Lavinia, taller than Lillian and with a slimmer waist, walked erect, head high with hair neatly arranged in a circular twist held in place with decorative pins. Lavinia had worked with Jane Delano, founder of the American Red Cross Nursing Service, during a yellow fever outbreak in Florida, and eventually was appointed as an administrator at Johns Hopkins School of Nursing. She was a commanding officer.

Having browsed her book superficially, Annette appreciated Lavinia's knowledge, heartened in knowing that nurses were now publishing books in their field. Seated next to Annette, Millie smiled when Lavinia was introduced. "I hope I never need her as my nurse," she whispered. Squelching laughter, Annette and Millie just managed to compose themselves.

Both women were intense, emanating passion for their profession and the public's health. Lillian's warm, welcoming approach contrasted with Lavinia's stern, dispiriting demeanor and clipped speech.

Each speaker provided an overview of her work, Lillian addressing ills of poverty, social welfare, and community health. She spoke of her experiences, some quite similar to Annette's home visit to Alice in Waltham, and the consequences of abject poverty and subsequent illness.

"We need to work together for the cause of human progress," Lillian advised, requesting that the club attend to *what is not seen, what is not known,* to the majority living in the Boston and Cambridge areas.

"Be willing to see and to know. With your help and openness to the public's poverty and misery, you will be loyal builders of healthy communities."

Hoping to stimulate conversation, Ellen asked how they might take up her cause.

"I advocate for awareness. Tour your cities. See tenements, walk the stairways, visit families, talk to Department of Health personnel. Once aware, you simply cannot turn away."

This was the first such call to action that club members had received. Requests for money, support letters, volunteer service, and other similar appeals had been logged previously, but this was different. Action, by members. A rather unheard-of request to Back Bay members.

Realizing that some would be, at the very least, reticent to embrace Lillian's unusual request, Ellen shifted attention quickly to Lavinia, to continue the group's conversations on suffrage. After thanking Lillian for her presentation, Ellen turned to Lavinia, introducing her as a political activist, and, at times, a militant suffragist.

"I have the luxury of wealth," she began, "as do many of you. I do not need to work for income, for food and housing. I work for women's causes, and to eradicate inequities." Lavinia strode the parlor room, stopping to look directly into members' eyes, purposely causing discomfort. Only wealthy women, she claimed, can ignore the right to vote. In describing a factory staffed with female workers at sewing machine stations in a crowded, poorly lit, dismal environment, Lavinia had concluded that only by voting would such workers have rights.

"As Frances Willard states, violence against women would cease if women had the right to vote. Frances has told me that she has presented to you recently. You know her arguments for suffrage. Have you been active in this effort?" Lavinia stood still, stating that her question was simply rhetorical. Most of the women looked down.

"Lillian and I both ask you to be active. Organized women are influencers. Spread the word, support suffrage, see poor people, walk through tenements, advocate for families' health." Lavinia noted that many among her own profession dismissed suffrage as a cause, believing voting efforts to be nonprofessional, perhaps crude, unladylike.

"How can intelligent women be so uninformed? So frightened by power?"

No one responded to Lavinia, and most eyes remained on the floor. As silence lengthened, Ellen moved to stand by Lillian and Lavinia, shaking their hands, thanking them for their presentations and calls for action.

Motioning to Millie to join her, Annette hurriedly walked toward Lillian and Lavinia, anticipating that Ellen would introduce them.

Gracious as always, Ellen introduced her niece and Millie. "Here," she said, "are ardent suffragists eager to further the cause and to recognize poverty and its consequences." As Ellen turned to talk to her crestfallen members, Annette and Millie were now alone with Lillian and Lavinia.

"Miss Wald," Annette began, "may I have a few minutes of your time before you leave?"

"Certainly," said Lillian. Lavinia looked on, eyebrows arched.

Millie approached Lavinia and, placing a hand on her forearm, drew her into a separate conversation about nursing textbooks, complimenting her on the success of her *Materia Medica for Nurses*. Millie had long ago learned to engage those above her with flattery from below.

On the opposite side of the parlor, Annette summarized for Lillian both her recent experiences at Waltham and her ongoing interest in nursing's education programs and scope of practice.

"I need to expand my observations. Would you please consider allowing Millie and me to observe the visiting nurse services you provide in New York City?" Taking in a deep breath, Annette hoped for a positive answer.

"It would be my pleasure to have you both join us as we provide services. Can you come this upcoming Saturday? We have several patient visits scheduled for this weekend."

"You work on weekends?"

Smiling gently at the privileged young woman before her, Lillian reassured Annette that health care and nursing were everyday activities, quite unlike most other endeavors. Hospitals, she added, offer every day, all day care, a major advantage for extremely ill patients. Since they did not have any examinations scheduled for Monday and their homework assignments could be completed quickly, Annette asked Lillian how early they might arrive. Annette jotted down the Jefferson Street address in her little notepad.

Thanking Lillian, Annette turned to Lavinia, who was explaining pharmacologic treatments to Millie. Annette caught the condescending tone of the older woman and knew, at once, how to handle one of her own. Annette asked Lavinia, while stepping between her and Millie, if she planned to attend the Chicago World's Fair later that year.

Drawing herself erect, with flat affect, Lavinia responded. "Of course, I shall attend. I am a leader in nursing." Miffed at being the second guest to be addressed, Lavinia described her close relationship with Isabel Hampton, the chairman of the subsection on nursing to be held during the International Congress of Charities, Correction and Philanthropy during the World's Fair.

"In 1890, I became the assistant superintendent of nursing at the Johns Hopkins School of Nursing, under Isabel Hampton's leadership. We have been colleagues and friends for several years now. I will be assisting her during the Nursing Congress." Clearly proud of her association with Isabel Hampton, Lavinia gestured dismissal of Annette and Millie by a hand wave as she walked to the front door.

"Miss Dock, we will also be attending the Nursing Congress. We will see you again in Chicago," said Annette. Annette intended to provoke.

Dock turned back. "But you are not a nurse," she said curtly, arms folded across her chest. "What could you possibly offer?"

"As an educated person interested in health care, I have much to offer," Annette snapped back. Returning to Millie and Ellen, Annette asked if they wished to continue discussing strategies on suffrage, well within earshot of Lavinia. The door closed behind her with a perceptible thud.

Yes, Annette thought, much to offer, and for many years to come.

"Rarely do I admit this, but I am too tired to talk. I must rest." Ellen hugged both women, leaving for her bedroom. Concerned for her aunt, Annette walked upstairs with her, quietly asking about her health. Ellen described an annoying cough and lethargy she had been experiencing for several weeks, now accompanied by occasional shortness of breath with even mild exertion. Annette suggested referral to Alfred, given that his specialty was pulmonary.

With Ellen's permission, Annette agreed to seek Alfred's counsel.

Even as Amos Fiske questioned the need for his presence at a meeting at Harvard called by Charles Eliot regarding the collegiate instruction of women, he was quite pleased to attend. His admiration for his alma mater was profound, as was his deepening respect for its current president. Caroline served as his valet, selecting a crimson-color necktie and matching handkerchief for his breast pocket. Wearing his frock coat, straight trousers, and Oxford shoes, Amos beamed at his wife, confidence growing to match his elegant appearance. Caroline asked why he had been summoned by Charles.

"Well, Caroline, I am a newsman with a legal background. Perhaps my blended skills may now come in handy." Amos knew that newspapers influenced readers, perhaps swaying them to support, or reject, proposed legislation. Amos realized that his zeal for his institution's efforts was not always objective. Gratitude for his education sometimes clouded rational thought. He had come to appreciate higher education for women only by recognizing his daughter Annette's growth as she sailed through classics at the Harvard Annex. Originally, he had not appreciated the need for women's education. It was only when he had moved his family to Cambridge for his son's Harvard education that he began to imagine his daughters as intellectual beings. As they matured, Amos realized their potential to contribute to society, their thirst for knowledge. Grateful that he and Caroline had enrolled their daughters at Arthur Gilman's Cambridge School for Girls, Amos was now a fervent supporter of the Annex, and he was hopeful that it would soon award academic degrees.

"Amos, you must know that I appreciate your support for the Annex, and for our daughters. I am simply not of their generation. I support women's right to vote, but I will remain in the background. And, while it is too late for me, education is important for women, for our daughters. Know also that I continue to want Annie and Margie to marry well, to have families and loving homes. I don't know if women can have all of these things, but I think it is important that they are given the opportunities to have it all."

Caroline, sitting in a chair in their dressing room, was awash with mixed feelings. The chair she sat in was comfortable and familiar, as was her home. But the world outside her home was changing too quickly for her. Ashamed of her jealousy of her daughters, Caroline saw her future opportunities as limited, as compared to the future now opening for them. She thought of her brother, a professor with a family, charming home, and interesting days filled with work he loved. The rhythms and routines of her life revolved around meals, laundry, and housework. She felt a twinge of resentment. *I will never be invited to participate in a meeting with Charles Eliot,* she thought.

Caroline wished Amos a successful meeting before returning to the kitchen to supervise preparations for dinner.

Dapper and confident, Amos joined Elizabeth Agassiz and Charles Eliot in the president's office at Harvard, eager to contribute to the conversation about women's education. Surprised by Charles's rather small mahogany desk and simple oil lamp, Amos was reminded of his humility, his drive for usefulness and appetite for details. Charles was about focus, not diffusion. They were here to set a plan in motion.

"We need to determine the steps necessary for the Annex to award diplomas for academic degrees, to be self-governing, to have a separate name from that of Harvard."

For now, Elizabeth suggested, let us simply refer to the Annex as *X College.* Charles and Amos agreed to the placeholder.

"We must be very clear on the history of X College, and so we must have an exact timeline of events," said Charles. With that, Elizabeth reviewed Arthur Gilman's conception of a program for private collegiate instruction for women, established by the Committee of Seven Lady Managers in 1879. Re-established as the Society for the Collegiate Instruction for Women in 1882, the executive committee, under Elizabeth's supervision and Charles's watchful presence, maintained focus on academic excellence and standards. Fay House, the current home of the Annex, facing Cambridge Commons from Garden Street, purchased in 1886, was described by Elizabeth as the first building of X College.

"We have been educating women for fourteen years, and our graduates have stellar academic records. Our efforts predict success as a degree-granting institution." She volunteered to write up the history.

When Elizabeth completed her review, Charles indicated that the next step was to understand the commonwealth's process for award of degree-granting authority. He described the process as straightforward, with drafting of a college charter as step one, followed by a hearing before the Committee on Education of the Massachusetts Legislature at the statehouse in Boston.

"The drafting of a college charter will be neither burdensome nor time-consuming, since we already have our Annex template," Charles said. "However," he continued, "I expect many objections to the endorsement of our final draft charter. Howls will come from many corners — members of the Harvard Board of Overseers and the Corporation, the fellows of the Harvard College, Harvard alumni, faculty of all our schools, our Back Bay community, legislators, and women themselves."

Glancing at Elizabeth, Charles commented that he had not always known women to be supportive of women. "Unfortunately," he continued, "I have witnessed this to be true, as have you."

"Remember also that legislators may see women's education as the first step to women's voting, anathema to many men." Charles, walking to face the fireplace, pointed to Amos.

"First, the vote. Then, prohibition," Charles said, smirking. "If women are educated, many will think that a step to perdition." He knew that an alternative narrative was needed, and he knew where one could be found.

"Amos, your role is critically important. You shape public opinion through the press. How do we present our efforts, manage dissent, and perhaps, even garner support?"

Understanding why he had been invited to the meeting, Amos immediately envisioned a five- or six-part series of weekly feature articles, printed below the fold on page one, on advancing education for women. *The Boston Globe,* founded in 1872, already enjoyed a reputation for prestigious investigative reporting. Competitive with *The New York Times,* founded in 1851, *The Globe* avoided sensationalism and muckraking, presenting objective facts to its readers. Women's education, a popular topic in the northeast region, would attract sophisticated, powerful readers, including legislators. Amos's plan for a series was well received by both Charles and Elizabeth.

Charles had a rolling blackboard brought into his office. Like generals detailing war strategies, Charles, Elizabeth, and Amos framed three columns, each relating to the main goal — award of degree-granting status to X College. In the first column, labeled *proponents,* were names of those thought to be in favor of the college. In the second, names of *opponents* of the college, with the third column reserved for names of influential people whose opinions on the subject were *unknown.*

"This chart is critical," said Charles. "We need to swing over the unknowns to the first column. It is highly unlikely we will sway diehard opponents. So, we must concentrate our efforts on the first and last columns, and therefore mitigate the impact of those in the second column." Over the next thirty minutes, they filled in the chart, adding names of individuals, groups, and organizations in the columns.

Names of the six sister colleges, the General Federation of Women Clubs, various legislators, notable Harvard alumni, the Massachusetts governor, religious organizations, Women's Christian Temperance Union, and others began to fill the chart.

"This is what we must anticipate," said Charles. "We need more advocates than opponents to swing the Committee on Education of our legislature. Elizabeth, what forces can you bring?"

Elizabeth paced as she spoke, jotting notes on the writing pad hanging from her waist.

"I'll organize meetings of current Annex students, as well as Annex alumni, to inform them of our goal and to listen to their objections, if any. Also, our goal will be the first action item on our next agenda of the Society. To have unanimous support, we need the endorsement of the seven women managers, as well as that of Arthur Gillman. I will ensure that our meeting minutes will record managers' votes." Elizabeth urged them to agree to the following statement as their goal: "The Society for the Collegiate Instruction of Women, otherwise called the Harvard Annex, is to be granted the authority to award diplomas for academic degrees, to be self-governing, and to have a separate name from that of Harvard."

Charles and Amos agreed to Elizabeth's bold wording, accepting it for use in all communications, meetings, newspaper articles, presentations, and any other forms for dissemination to the public.

Amos thought it would work well in *The Globe* series, perhaps as a lead to the second article once the stage was set with the first advocating the advantages of women's education.

"With you, Elizabeth, I'll meet with the Harvard Corporation and the overseers, securing their approval of our goal. While they will certainly have questions about finances, I do believe I have a possible avenue for a new endowment. Matthew Campbell, a recent appointment to the Harvard Board of Overseers, plans to endow a professorship of arts to Harvard. He is very fond of Annette and Amos. With Annette our model, it is very possible that we may convince him to endow X College as a whole, rather than simply the arts, a much broader gift within the Harvard community."

The Harvard alumni, Charles knew, were historically disagreeable to any change. The topic of educating women might seem a violation of their very dignity, utterly unimaginable, absurd. Viewing women biblically as sources of enticement and evil, alumni might rather close Harvard itself than see it ravaged by the presence of women. It would seem a deeply flawed financial investment. These views, however, primarily marked older alumni, those graduating prior to his presidency under a more restricted canvas. Younger alumni, trained in sciences, engineering, modern languages, and other subjects, would be more open to having a sister college award degrees to women.

"I will speak also to the alumni and to the general faculty. The faculty minutes will reflect outcomes of discussions and, hopefully, endorsement of our goal."

"One final thought," said Charles. "We would do well to invite Alfred Worcester and his wife, Elizabeth, to speak with the faculty, especially the medical and dental school faculty. As I have seen quite recently, Alfred has a very winning, congenial way of influencing people. And Elizabeth, the daughter of Thomas Hill, who preceded me as Harvard's president, has a calming demeanor, one reminiscent of her father's soothing presence. Elizabeth might help our cause with the older faculty." Elizabeth Agassi and Amos, who enjoyed Alfred's enthusiasm for education and loyalty to Harvard, believed Charles's suggestion a great one, asking him to speak with Alfred as soon as possible.

Eternally summarizing, Charles jotted their agreements on the blackboard to maintain focus and determine next actions. Having agreed on the goal, each had homework. Each realized that assignments needed to be completed before next steps could be undertaken. The next meeting of the larger core planning group, including Alfred, Annette, and Millie, had already been scheduled for an upcoming Monday morning.

As Amos and Elizabeth prepared to leave, Charles surprised them by returning to the subject of a name for the college.

"All institutions have names. What shall we call the Annex?" Charles offered Emmanuel College, the institution that John Harvard graduated from in 1632 and 1635, with baccalaureate and master's degrees, respectively. Both Elizabeth and Amos frowned at this suggestion, thinking that X College need not be named after a man.

"Charles, do you recall the first endowed scholarship at Harvard donated by Lady Mowlson, an English entrepreneur active in Puritan causes?" Elizabeth noted that Lady Mowlson, whose maiden name was Ann Radcliffe, gave Harvard one hundred pounds in 1643 for a scholarship, with, as she put it, "revenue from it to be employed that way forever." Suggesting that Radcliffe was an appropriate name for X College, given its picturesqueness and history as the name of the first female benefactor to Harvard, Elizabeth championed it. The two men agreed.

Their idea had a name: Radcliffe College.

At 6:30 am, the sun was rising in the east over the North Union Station on Causeway Street, Boston, as Annette and Millie, dressed in winter garb, waited for their New York, New Haven, and Hartford train to arrive. Still under construction, the North Station was impressive, wind howling through incomplete sections of the building. The station's central triumphal arch, bordered by two Ionic columns, reminded Annette of Greek architecture, with its three orders of design style serving as both art and structural support. Ever pleased that ancient Greek architecture continued to influence the modern era, Annette relaxed in the large, airy waiting room. She was aware that her life in Cambridge — insular, encompassing a distance of no more than one mile between Fay House to her home at 1564 Massachusetts Avenue — was about to expand by rail.

The world beyond her life was moving fast, Annette realized, as she watched work crews hauling building materials and railroad personnel carrying office furniture hustle quickly between completed sections of the station and those still under construction. Up to now, she thought, her world had been secure, pleasant, comforting, and predictable. Now she was enmeshed in a noisy cyclone of energy, dynamic, unpatterned. Even the railroad line, popularly called the New Haven, had only acquired the New York, Providence, and Boston Railroad one year earlier, providing commuters with expanded service on the northeast corridor, with the Pennsylvania Railroad Station at Paulus Hook, Jersey City, as the final terminal. From Boston to Jersey City, New Jersey, the trip would cover approximately 220 miles, with planned stops along the journey. At the Paulus Hook terminal station on the western shore of North River, they would transfer to a ferry, cross the river, and arrive at the Cortland Street Ferry Depot in lower Manhattan, home to Lillian Wald.

For Annette, the trip was a return to her roots. While born in Massachusetts, she lived as a young child in New York City, in a first-floor apartment on Mercer Street, neighboring Washington Square Park and New York University. While her father had accepted a position at *The Boston Globe* when the family moved to Cambridge, he retained membership in New York's Century Association, a private club for men known for distinction in literature, that he had joined when he worked for *The New York Times*. The clubhouse was located on Broadway in Lower Manhattan, on the periphery of the Lower East Side. Since Annette's memories of her New York childhood centered on her family's home, she was surprised by her father's description of the Lower East Side, the section of the city where she and Millie were to spend a week with Lillian.

When she told her father of her visit, his description of poverty among immigrant families was a stark contrast to memories of her affluent neighborhood. The Lower East Side, as he described it, was a vibrant, crowded, busy section of the city. He noted that the area primarily now housed Russian and Eastern European immigrants of Jewish descent, many of whom had escaped pogroms in their native countries. Orchard Street, about eight blocks between Chinatown and East Houston Street on the Lower East Side, is lined with tenement buildings, he noted, many with five to seven floors of low-income, 325-square-foot apartments, most with three rooms.

"Tenement fire escapes," Amos had continued, "characterize these buildings. Large families expand their living space by using fire escapes for drying clothes, storage, and simply relaxing." Escaping hatred in their native countries, Jewish immigrants worked long hours in low-paying jobs and lived in crowded tenements, subject to infectious diseases and industrial injuries. He stressed, however, that the neighborhoods of the Lower East Side offered freedom to Jewish immigrants, as they had for German immigrants in previous generations, with storefront synagogues fashioned in tenement parlors and kosher Jewish foods offered in open-air marketplaces. America offered hope.

Annette asked her father if he knew anything of Jefferson Street, where Lillian lived.

"Ah," he said. "Lillian lives in the heart of the Lower East Side. I imagine that she is kept busy with the health needs of her community. Jacob Riis has documented conditions of families living in poverty in the Lower East Side."

"From what Charlotte Macleod has said of her," Annette added, "Lillian comes from a wealthy Jewish family currently living in Ohio. Her uncle, Henry, a medical doctor trained in Vienna, began a surgical program at Columbia University just a decade ago." Having only a brief sketch of Lillian from Charlotte, Annette described a class on home nursing care she offered to immigrant families at the Hebrew Technical School for Girls, shortly after brief employment at the New York Juvenile Asylum orphanage.

"After caring for a young woman who had hemorrhaged in childbirth," Annette continued, "Lillian resolved to live in the Lower East Side to give direct care to poor families. In an apartment on Jefferson Street, she and her friend Mary Brewster started nursing services in their new community."

As the boarding call rang out for those travelling to Jersey City, Annette rallied from her recollected conversation with her father. Knowing that they would be quite busy while in New York, she and Millie decided to catch up on coursework. Annette opened her copy of *Oedipus Tyrannus* as Millie began her translation of *Antigone*. Against the gentle rumbling of the train, Sophocles did not stand a chance. They both fell fast asleep. Finding them angelic, the conductor paused before telling them that they had arrived at their destination.

Despite blustery cold breezes and threatening gray sky, Annette and Millie chose seats on the upper deck of the ferry *New Brunswick* at the Pennsylvania Railroad Station in Jersey City. They wanted to see everything.

After paying a nickel each, they huddled snugly in wooden folding chairs with hands firmly planted on the ferry's outer guardrail, sailing the North River for fourteen minutes before reaching the Cortland Street Ferry Depot in New York City. Like the North Union Station in Boston, the seven-story Pennsylvania Railroad Station terminal at Paulus Hook had been reconstructed in 1892, with a large arched roof, four elevators called tubes, and multiple waiting areas for passengers. The terminal's architect, Charles Schneider, claimed it the largest terminal in the United States.

All new, all exciting to Annette and Millie. Indeed, a modern world.

Upon disembarking at Cortland Street Ferry Depot, their trip became more adventuresome, beginning with a short eight-seat passenger horse-drawn carriage ride to a trolley stop on Broadway, and from there, to a Manhattan Elevated Railroad at Canal Street, traveling to East Broadway. Weary, but still enthusiastic, Annette and Millie disembarked on East Broadway, having decided to walk the remaining distance to Jefferson Street. Their five-minute walk took them to Jefferson Street first through Henry Street, and then Madison Street, a neighborhood core to Lillian's catchment area.

Lillian's neighborhood is as my father described, thought Annette, absorbing sights of multiple-story tenement buildings with prominent fire escapes and throngs of people crowding packed-dirt streets. Carriage after carriage displaying fruits, vegetables, and other produce were parked at the edges of streets, jammed against each other, with owners encouraging passersby to buy their fresh foods. Some carriages were sheltered by large canvas umbrellas providing coverage for their produce, many with names written in Hebrew.

While Annette saw the streets and buildings, Millie saw people, particularly children, girls with long curls in loose dresses belted with sashes and boys with knickerbockers and hand-me-down bonnets from their fathers. Millie saw children playing happily in the streets with large hoops and cups and balls on sticks, mingling among adults and food carriages. Several carriages were managed by Hasidic men with side curls, or payot, identifying them as members of the Orthodox Jewish community. While yarmulkes were usually worn during prayer time or holy events, Millie noted that a few men, and several women, were wearing them as they walked through the street markets.

Their bright-green and brown wool work carpetbags becoming heavy and cumbersome, Annette and Millie were relieved upon seeing the sign for Jefferson Street.

It was now four o'clock in the afternoon, and they were hungry, having finished the last apples and bananas stashed in their bags. During their brief walk from East Broadway to Lillian's tenement on Jefferson, the aromas arising from the food trucks tantalized them, teasing them to enjoy knishes or macaroons. Since they did not know if Lillian had any plans for dinner, they practiced discipline, walking quickly past the trucks to avoid temptation.

They found a note from Lillian on her apartment door.

"A family on Henry Street has asked for my assistance. I shall return as quickly as possible. Please ask Tommie, the young boy living with his mother in the basement, for the key to my apartment. I shall see you soon. I have dinner ready for us. Lillian"

Carpetbags in hand, Annette and Millie walked the five flights of stairs from the fourth floor to the basement, keenly aware of the increasing dinginess and musky odor as they descended. A small piece of paper with the word *Janitress* handwritten on it was tacked to a door in the basement with hide glue.

Tommie, eight years old, wore baggy trousers, a small man's jacket with missing buttons, and an oversized soft, rounded cap with a stiff bill and central button on the crown. With smudged face, soiled hands, and warm smile, he greeted them enthusiastically.

"Pleased to meet you," Tommie said, extending his arm for handshakes. "I'm happy to take you to the ladies' rooms," he beamed, almost running up the staircase.

"I like to help the ladies," said Tommie, smiling from ear to ear. "They live like the Queen of England and eat off of solid gold plates." Tommie and Lillian had bonded quickly, he helping with minor chores in exchange for dinners at her table.

Meticulously neat, Lillian's apartment had four rooms, including a small sitting parlor, one bedroom with a double bed, and a dining room connected to a kitchen. The fire escape, available from the kitchen, held several large boxes, apparently serving as storage space. The kitchen contained both a bathtub and a stove, with a spigot for water in the hall. The floors, painted brown, were covered with thin beige carpets, and the windows curtained with bright scrim, providing privacy as well as a sunscreen. The bathroom, at the end of the hallway, was communal, with the additional option of using an outhouse or privy.

On the fifth floor, the apartment's fire escape opened to the tenement's roof, allowing, according to Lillian, an easy route for jumping from tenement to tenement on busy days. Looking at the fire escapes, Annette secretly hoped that she and Millie would experience crossing among tenements with Lillian, hopping roof to roof. She and Millie wanted to experience it all.

Tommie placed an old mattress on the floor in the bedroom, telling them that Lillian would sleep there, and they would both sleep in the bed. "Mary," he explained, "is gone to visit her family for a few days, so you are lucky to have the bed."

"The ladies work every day. My mum, Mrs. McRae, and me live in the basement. She is the janitress for the building, and she helps the ladies too when they need it. My mum protects them. They have lots of visitors, and we make sure they don't hurt the ladies."

Tommie led them to the kitchen of Lillian's apartment, where a large pot of soup with carrots, celery, basil, chicken, and matzo balls remained on the stove, the delightful smell wafting through the room. Annette noticed a bottle of concord grape wine on the small square table, surrounded by three glasses.

Lillian returned at sunset, eager to serve her guests dinner and to describe the nursing work that she and Mary had begun on Jefferson Street.

As she took off her full-length dark-brown cloak, gloves, and small brimmed hat, Lillian reviewed her work to her guests.

"As you know from our last meeting, Mary and I call our work public health nursing. That comes down to keeping families healthy. Mary and I help residents to eat well, to manage illness, to care for children and older parents, to be responsible for themselves." Lillian described her neighborhood as home to Jewish Russian and Polish immigrants who needed to learn English, to become citizens, to hold jobs, and to be free to practice their religion.

"There is much work to be done, but our nursing schools focus on doctors' orders, not patient health or home care. Pupil nurses are the equipment of hospitals."

Fearful that nursing was becoming captivated with the allure of hospital care to the disadvantage of home care, Lillian praised Annette's description of the clinical training in homes and at industrial sites offered by the Waltham Training School for Nurses. The three women spoke long into the night, with Annette and Millie absorbing Lillian's stories and advice for expanded health and social services in industrial cities. As Lillian described the accidents and injuries common in the garment industry, Annette began to appreciate the similarities between and among settings as diverse as Waltham and the Lower East Side. Again, she thought of her father's descriptions, Jacob Riis's book, Charlotte Macleod's worries, and now, Lillian's work.

Yes, Annette thought, there is much, so much, to be done.

Lillian retreated to the bedroom, eager to end her long day. Wishing them a good night, she blew out her candle, leaving Annette and Millie in the kitchen. Intrigued by the fire escape, they opened the window, settling on the landing.

Millie passed a cigarette to Annette as they sat on the fire escape reviewing their day. Legs dangling off the fire escape, their silence was unusual. The sheer magnitude and complexity of Lillian's efforts, too elusive to grasp, rendered them silent.

After a few minutes, Millie wandered back to Hippocrates's *On Airs, Waters, Places*, something that was familiar. She recalled his recognition of the mutual interaction between man and environment, as well as the development of illness resulting from imbalance between the two.

"There is," she said, "an imbalance here. Not being sick does not mean that a person is healthy. The science of health is as important as the science of disease."

They agreed that their next report to the Cambridge group must persuade the team that nursing was a lead player in ensuring peoples' health. Annette and Millie knew their arguments must be convincing, based on objective findings, all within the context of the progress sweeping the country. They realized just how important their visit to New York was becoming.

Annette and Millie spent their first night in Lillian's apartment sleepless. They had gone to bed late, and the next day promised to be complex, with two home visits and a scheduled trip to a potential benefactor. Wondering if they had the energy to follow Lillian's life, both Annette and Millie realized that they were incredibly drawn to it. The sheer potential to contribute to improving peoples' lives was overwhelmingly attractive.

Over breakfast at her kitchen table, Lillian explained that Jacob Schiff was a Jewish banker born in Germany in 1847 who now lived in Manhattan on Fifth Avenue. She described Jacob as a philanthropist abhorring antisemitism, and passionate about the Jewish principle of Zedakah, or the ethical obligation to do what is right. As news of Lillian and Mary's work circulated within the Russian-Jewish community on the Lower East Side, Jacob's interest in their efforts peaked. Keenly aware of the poverty and illness rampant in those neighborhoods, Jacob knew that the Eastern Dispensary, or the Good Samaritan Dispensary as referred to by local residents, at 75 Essex Street on the corner of Essex and Broome Streets, was overwhelmed by patient volume.

Jacob had visited the dispensary only two years ago, seeing the diverse patient population in the large waiting room seeking care. Listless babies in their mothers' arms, young men with broken arms in slings or broken legs supported by makeshift crutches, frail older couples sitting quietly with bowed heads and crossed hands, and pregnant women with drawn, pale faces. As America hospitalized, Jacob had thought, the poor had been left behind to suffer.

He recognized that services provided by Lillian and Mary were desperately needed.

Jacob scheduled a meeting with them at 265 Henry Street in the Lower East Side to explore their community health services. His meeting coincided with Annette and Millie's visit.

If they cared for Russian Jewish immigrants, and he hoped that they did, then Jacob intended to fund their efforts within the Talmudic principle of *twice blessed is he who gives in secret*. As they took their seats in a small, unfurnished room in the Henry

Street apartment, Jacob congratulated Lillian on her work, voicing disappointment at not meeting Mary Brewster. He was, however, interested in learning of Annette and Millie's interest in Lillian's public health nursing services. He was equally intrigued by their academic pursuits, querying them on their reasons to visit Lillian and the Lower East Side more generally. Annette provided a summary of the goals of the Cambridge planning group, with Millie expanding on the broad goal to establish a Harvard school of nursing.

"Any academic nursing school must focus on health, modeled conceptually on the services being offered here, within the Lower East Side," stressed Annette. Annette worried that perhaps she had overstepped her description to a New York banker she hardly knew.

To Annette's surprise, Jacob smiled at her comment.

"Yes," Jacob, leaning toward Annette, said that he agreed with her and Millie's statements. "Harvard, nursing, health. This is an excellent combination, one incredibly needed at this time. I am glad that your president, Charles Eliot, has the wisdom to predict the value of such a school."

Returning to Lillian, Jacob sought her advice on what she needed to expand her services.

"A place, Mr. Schiff. We need a home, a settlement to ground our work." Lillian described her burgeoning patient population, the materials needed to provide home care, public health bags, the educational resources vital for teaching health, among other items. We need storage. Smiling, she indicated that her fire escape doubled as office storage. Stressing the need for patient documentation and storage of health records, Lillian aroused Jacob's keen interest in efficient administration.

Jacob promised to investigate a new location for Lillian's visiting nurse services, including possible expansion to a building on Henry Street.

"If a building you deem appropriate becomes available on Henry Street, then would you consider relocation? Such a building could be renovated for patient services as well as offering you and Mary safe housing."

"Selecting and refurbishing an appropriate building will take time, so in the meantime I might be able to support several of your needs. What are your thoughts, Lillian?"

Jacob, calmly smoothing his well-trimmed white beard with his left hand, slowly positioned his ink pen and stationery on his leather desk blotter, as if to write a letter. For a moment, Lillian was unable to speak. Recovering, she then thanked Jacob for his generosity.

The meeting concluded, Jacob shook hands with the three women and wished them well in their efforts.

Outside the building, the women lingered at the corner of Henry and Montgomery Streets.

"We must talk tonight, after dinner," said Lillian, looking at her watch, realizing that the meeting was longer than she expected, delaying her family visits. There was no celebration, no moment of reflection. There was only the work. Leaving them on the corner, Lillian rushed off to those who needed her.

She was, Annette and Millie knew, a marvel.

Over the next three days, Annette and Millie joined Lillian on her visits. Keeping pace with her was not an easy task. Fast walks, stair climbing, and zigzagging between people, food carriages, and horses taxed Lillian's guests.

Annette's desire to jump from tenement roof to tenement roof, used as a time-saving strategy, was realized. After climbing to the top floor of one building, then crawling out the kitchen window to the fire escape landing and then onto the roof, Annette paled as she looked at the one-foot distance to the next building. Lillian does this frequently, she thought. Adjusting her bloomers and short skirt, Annette glanced at Millie, nodding to jump together.

During those days, Annette and Millie became proud of their stamina and ability to match, however haltingly, Lillian's endurance. Competitive, Annette was determined to remain at Lillian's side. Grateful that she and Millie had taken Lillian's advice and worn bloomers with shortened skirts, in future trips she would replace her low-heel lace-up Balmoral boots with more sensible low-heel walking shoes. Not accustomed to sustained physical effort, Annette promised to exercise more frequently.

"Our next visit is to a very poor young family living in a third-floor apartment in a tenement on Henry Street. Their one-month-old baby is having difficulty breastfeeding. She is not thriving and has lost a pound from her birth weight. The mother is depressed, and her milk flow is decreasing. The other children seem well, but undernourished." Lillian described the baby's father as a garment worker who spent ten-hour shifts at Harris Levine's apartment at 97 Orchard Street, where Harris had established a small, but competitive garment shop. The father, only home on Saturdays to observe the Sabbath, was unable to spend much time with his family.

Lillian's examination of the newborn confirmed that she was failing to thrive and unable to latch onto her mother's breast to feed. Knowing that the Eastern Dispensary on Essex Street would not assist in this case, she asked the mother if a *landsmanshafn*, an organization of Jewish families, operated in her neighborhood. Since she was aware of such a group on her block, Lillian encouraged the mother to seek their help in securing a wet nurse, and, if breastfeeding continued to be too difficult, to begin bottle feeding with animal's milk and to offer panada, made by boiling bread in water and then combining the paste with egg yolks or butter and given as a supplement by pap-boat shallow vessel with a lip for feeding young children. She also suggested that the local *landsmanshafn* might have fruit that could be given to the other children.

By their last home visit on the third day, all three women were anxious for the Sabbath, Saturday, the accepted day of rest.

"You will enjoy our last day together. As Annex students, you will be in your element," Lillian smiled. She explained that they would visit the Hebrew Technical School for Girls, at 240 Second Avenue. Now thirteen years old, the school had two divisions. One assisted girls for jobs in commerce and industry, while the second prepared girls for positions in the dressmaking and millinery sector.

Lillian said that they would instruct dressmaking students on basic feminine hygiene, including sex education, the birthing process, and types of sexually transmitted diseases. The visit required a short carriage ride from Henry Street to Second Avenue, a little more than a mile away. Quiet observers to the session, Annette and Millie were impressed by the frank conversations, direct questions, and quest for additional information on the part of the students, all young teenage girls preparing for entry into the garment business.

Lillian left the students with a final message: "Take care of yourselves. Remember that you are the most important person to you."

Later that afternoon, Lillian, Annette, and Millie reviewed their conversation with Jacob Schiff. Jacob's funding would be crucial to Lillian's continued work in the community. Lillian only discussed finances on their last day, revealing that she charged either no payment or very little payment for her services. Funding would enable expansion, possible recruitment of more nursing staff, and health supplies. Noting that a gift to a new Harvard school of nursing would also be outstanding, Lillian hinted that remaining faithful to teaching health rather than simply assisting in managing disease would be important to Jacob's mission.

Then she was off again, for one last home visit, as night fell on Jefferson Street.

At seven o'clock the next morning, after a long goodbye to Lillian, Annette and Millie started home, taking the Manhattan Elevated Railroad on East Broadway to Canal Street, then to Broadway by trolley, and finally to the Cortland Street Ferry Depot. Through Lillian's eyes, Annette saw families of homeless people living in tents under the elevated railroad. She knew what she must do.

Exhilaration

"Breathtaking! Glorious! Brilliant!"

As the sun set on Sunday, June 11, 1893, Alistair Campbell, like his three colleagues, was stunned by the sudden brilliance of millions of Westinghouse stopper lamps illuminating the White City and the Court of Honor at the Chicago Columbian Exposition. The golden dome of the Administration Building and facades of structures within the fair's White City sparkled, and an extensive network of streetlights enabled fairgoers to roam long into the evening among the nearly two hundred temporary buildings of neoclassical architecture.

Standing outside the Administration Building, Alistair glanced at the Electricity Building to his left. While a banker, Alistair had always been intrigued with electricity, finding himself drawn to both the power and the beauty of light. Prior to the trip, he had read that the exposition was energized by twelve one-thousand-horsepower alternating current generators designed by Nikola Tesla, a Serbian-American engineer who participated in the 1893 fair at the invitation of Westinghouse Electric.

How gifted, how ingenious Tesla is, thought Alistair. He realized that Tesla, just thirty-seven years old, about the same age as Alfred Worcester standing next to him, had radically changed everything.

On May 1, 1893, opening day of the exposition, President Grover Cleveland had pressed the gold button wired in Washington to electrify the fair. The button was at the top of a three-tiered pyramid on a ceremonial table, with the dates 1492–1893 painted in silver on the bottom tier. One gesture, and the night had vanished. The world was filled with light. The world had changed forever.

Browsing through the *Official Guide to the World's Columbian Exposition*, Alistair was quite surprised that Tesla was not acknowledged by name, despite his personal display housed at the Westinghouse Company exhibit, the company responsible for incandescent lighting and special power. An oversight? he wondered. Ever a banker, Alistair saw the commercial value of Tesla's inventiveness. Perhaps there was some complexity in the scientist himself that would not square with the fair's narrative of unfettered progress.

On this balmy, warm June evening, however, Alistair was delighted to be at the fair.

"Do any of you want to join me for a quick visit to the Electricity Building?" Alistair asked Annette, Millie, and Alfred.

"As enchanting as your invitation sounds, Alistair," said Annette, "I am quite eager to locate the Art Building, where we must be tomorrow morning by ten." Considered private individuals and not official members of the Congress, she and her colleagues, upon the recommendation of Charles Eliot, had been especially endorsed by Henry M. Hurd, superintendent of Johns Hopkins Hospital and secretary of Section III of the International Congress of Charities, Correction, and Philanthropy, to attend sessions consistent with their interests. Fearful of being dismissed at the front door, Annette hoped to be first in line for admission, giving herself time to argue for a seat in the room if necessary. Hopefully, she thought, Charles's influence would prevail, and they would be able to attend the opening session tomorrow as well as other conferences on nurse training and hospital care of the sick without incident.

"Alistair, I'll go to the Electricity Building with you," said Millie. Annette and Alfred agreed to roam the fair for the Art Building, several buildings west of the Court of Honor, as Alistair and Millie headed directly to the Electricity Building, cited in the guidebook as "the most novel and brilliant of the exhibits."

Disappointed by the *CLOSED* sign on the Electricity Building, Alistair was too excited to turn back to their hotel. He suggested they do something entirely different, something particularly unusual.

"Let's take a ride in a Venetian gondola and sail through the Grand Basin and Lagoon. The Italian gondolier looks authentic enough." Besides, the gondolier's red-striped shirt and straw hat, worn at a jaunty angle, were reasons to linger a bit longer at the fair.

"Absolutely!" Millie, assisted by Alistair and the gondolier, climbed into the swan gondola. Alistair paid the fifty cents round-trip ticket.

"Tell me, Millie, what is your role in this game headed by Charles Eliot?" Alistair, a mischievous gleam in his eyes, smirked at Millie. He was in high spirits and found that this little boat ride might allow him to decipher Millie's role in what he thought of as *Annette's Adventure.*

"Why, dear Alistair, I am in Charles's game to advance women."

With concrete, unabashed conviction, Millie described her abhorrence of the treatment of women in America. "Education," she claimed, "is the key to being seen, to being heard." Education would eradicate invisibility, enabling women to contribute meaningfully, beyond reproduction. Radcliffe must be degree-granting. And Harvard must soon admit women. Perhaps, she offered, nursing may be the single best vehicle to effect change.

"As long as Charles Eliot promotes nursing as a degree offering at Harvard, I will be crew for him."

"And you, Alistair, why are you at the World's Fair as a part of this?" asked Millie.

"That's an easy one, Millie," Alistair said. Apart from enjoying the companionship of the group, he was loyal to Harvard, and to its president. Both Alistair and his father, Matthew, understood their talent for finance, appreciating that their knowledge was an asset to their alma mater. While his father had originally thought to endow an arts program at Harvard, both he and Alistair were now reconsidering, toying seriously with the establishment of a Harvard endowment in nursing. Such an endowment would secure a firm footing for a new school, recognizing the credibility of nursing as a major health profession.

"So I am here at the bow, in order to secure nursing's financial future at Harvard, perhaps by the turn of the century."

"But," he laughed, "I am also here because I like a fair." They both looked at the gondolier and his biceps. "You see, Millie, with you, I am a fan of endowments."

"There is so much to see — and to admire."

Giggling together as they looked up at the gondolier, they composed themselves as they realized the gondolier was scowling at them both.

Clearing his throat to begin the conversation again along more serious lines, Alistair asked Millie if she planned to become a nurse. Emphatically, Millie said no, that she lived in, and loved, her ancient world and wished to become an expert in it. She added, however, that she realized that both the past and present are fueled by effective administration. To achieve their goals, the Eliot group needed at least one member to understand facets of administration, to truly appreciate the nuances in managing people as well as money. A Harvard school of nursing would require detailed management for recruitment, marketing, building, finances, students, faculty, and other relevant features.

"Including endowments," she added, with a wink, "from handsome young men who just happen to be wealthy."

She wanted to gain proficiency, and to contribute, in academic administration. Better that, she thought, than spend a lifetime passing our syllabi to those who cared little about a world she loved.

"I do my own laundry and cook my food. I understand the details of daily life. You are an expert in finances. Charles needs both of us."

Alistair proposed a game. "Let us imagine that we are a rowing crew of eight, a merry band all pulling together. How shall we arrange ourselves in our Cambridge rowing shell?"

Like clever children apart from the world, they warmed to the game. The stern pair leading the boat would be Annette and Alfred, the most competitive of the crew. Annette would set the timing, and Alfred would be the buffer between her and the rest of the crew. The middle crew, the engines, would be Annette's Aunt Ellen and Stubby, as well as Amos and Caroline. They would pull the shell along. Millie and Alistair, both decided of themselves, would be the couple in the bow, giving calls to the crew and providing the necessary stability. As they recognized of each other, both were equally quick and, if necessary, could adapt to the boat's pitching—even anticipate it—in a moment's notice.

"And what of Charles?" Millie asked.

Smirking, Alistair sat up straight and declared, "Why, who else for the coxswain but Charles?"

They both burst into laughter again as the gondolier, singing a romantic song in Italian as their short trip ended, helped them exit the gondola, pointing them in the direction of their hotel. Alistair tipped him handsomely.

Gazing at the same sunset at the extreme west of the Court of Honor, Annette and Alfred stood on the grand steps of the Grecian-Ionic styled Art Building at the intersection of Michigan Avenue and Adams Street. The doorman and guards referred to it as the Art Palace. The only windowless structure in the exposition, the palace's ceilings, external colonnade and pillars, loggias, nave, and broad transept, were built to highlight paintings, sculptures, and statues.

Constructed in 1893 to replace the original Chicago Academy of Fine Arts erected in 1879, the Art Palace would serve as home to the world's congresses convening during the exposition, with thirty-three meeting halls each accommodating from one hundred to seven hundred attendees, six committee rooms, and two large audience rooms each with capacity of three thousand attendees. The building could hold thirty-six large meetings and over three hundred sectional meetings in a single week.

Looking up at the two temporary plaster-cast lions perched on the north and south ends of the Art Building, Alfred felt powerful. Annette wondered if he might be suppressing an urge to roar. At his side, she, too, glowed confidence as she absorbed the lions. So symbolic, she thought, of august new beginnings, a new era. The fair imaged America as the world's compelling leader, and, in doing so, the atmosphere instilled energy in individuals to lead, to surpass previous accomplishments. Surely, the organizers had imagined that the new world to come would be the American century.

We are going to be part of this, Annette thought, glancing at Alfred by her side.

"Tomorrow, Alfred, I would like to tour the Art Building, after the morning address by Reverend Peabody. My colleagues at the Annex say that the sculptures by the White Rabbits are quite beautiful."

"White Rabbits?" Alfred asked.

As they retraced their steps from the Art Building to the Women's Building on their return to the Columbian Central Hotel at Sixty-Second Street and Stony Island Avenue, Annette described the White Rabbits, female sculptors hired by the fair's chief architect, Daniel Burnham, to hurriedly create full-scale sculptures from small models sent by artists. Laughing, Annette noted that Burnham was reported to have told his staff to hire anyone, even white rabbits if they'll work.

"Women, Alfred," quipped Annette, "always get the job done."

Despite their daylong journey from Boston, they were far from tired. Alfred and his wife, Elizabeth, had recently returned from Europe, where they had visited hospitals and training schools for nurses in Great Britain, Switzerland, and Germany to learn best approaches to care of patients. He told Annette about that trip, with more attention to how that time away had allowed them to recover following the realization that they would be childless. Annette was truly pleased, she told Alfred, that the trip abroad had allowed them to find a path from their sadness.

Eager to see more, Alfred and Annette decided to visit the Midway Plaisance before retiring, particularly given the excellent lighting along the route connecting the fair's White City in Jackson Park to Washington Park in the west. After paying a fee, they exited the subway and entered the midway, a one-mile-long entertainment carnival of rides, food concessions, and exotic exhibits, designed to titillate visitors, encouraging them to purchase souvenirs and ride tickets. Central to the midway was the Ferris wheel, a 264-foot structure capable of accommodating 2,160 passengers per ride, costing fifty cents for a two-revolution trip.

Annette and Alfred walked briskly toward the Ferris wheel, thrilled for a seat in this lauded attraction, built to compete with the 1889 Paris Exposition's Eiffel Tower. As they approached the location, they realized they were ten days too early, given its targeted opening date of June 21st. Undaunted, they strolled briskly past entrances to many anthropological exhibits.

Unlike the buildings of the White City, particularly the Anthropology Building designed by Frederic W. Putnam, curator of the Peabody Museum of Archaeology and Ethnology at Harvard University, the midway exhibits seemed to Annette and Alfred to be arranged in a type of social Darwinian order. In order of appearance, the buildings descended from cultures similar to White Americans downward to those more unlike them, including the West African Dahomeans and Indigenous Americans among the last exhibits. Vaguely uneasy reading circus-like exhibit advertisements aimed to profit from people described as native savages in indigenous costumes, Annette and Alfred returned to the subway, and from there, to their hotel.

"Alfred, is this who we are? Displaying cultures dissimilar to our own as savages?" She wondered how the residents in the Lower East Side would be described at the midway.

"No," answered Alfred, "this is capitalism and only part, not the whole, of what we are. The midway is designed to make money. Perhaps more than the White City." As Alfred took her hand to guide her on the hotel steps, Annette realized that his grip remained just a heartbeat too long.

Alfred dropped her hand, saying in a low tone, head bowed, "I apologize, Annette. Our day has been long, and I seem to have forgotten my manners."

"No need to apologize, Alfred," Annette responded, looking into his eyes. "I have had a lovely day."

They ascended the steps, wished each other a good evening, and went, separately, to their own rooms.

Surprised at her own exhaustion, Annette admitted that she was happy to return to the room she and Millie shared at the Columbian Central Hotel. Only one block west of the central gate of the exposition, the location was ideal. For a one-week stay, the cost was one dollar each per day to share a room. Since the hotel had only three hundred rooms, she was grateful that Elizabeth Agassiz had recommended booking rooms in early spring.

Understanding Millie's finances, Elizabeth had also suggested that she serve as the Annex's representative. Elizabeth provided Millie with discretionary income to fund her expenses for a week. She also encouraged Millie to peruse her student wardrobe closet to select items that would augment her travel clothing.

"You need not look like you are always on your way to a seminar," Elizabeth had advised.

Millie entered the room, and she and Annette shared their stories of gondola games and midway exhibits. They emptied their large carpetbags and prepared for sleep, looking forward to the first day of the International Congress convention the next day. Annette set her adjustable alarm clock to 7:00 am, glad that her father had given it to her for the trip, knowing that she was a perfectionist detesting tardiness. Millie admired the leather case that held it and aimed to save for one like it.

"This is our second major trip in one year," Millie said from her bed. "We are gathering information more quickly than I had imagined."

Annette nodded agreement. "We'll need to condense our information, make it manageable for — what did you call it? — the crew to digest, once home. Our next planning meeting will be very important. Perhaps we can review our information during our train ride home."

Millie then told Annette more about their places in the shell, decided with Alistair. Annette loved the idea and decided that the little team would now be a Harvard crew.

"According to my souvenir edition guidebook," Alfred said the next morning, as he ran his fingers over the stiff cloth and gilded top of his one-dollar edition, "we can purchase a glass of Hygeia Waukesha water for one cent at any of several concessions at the park." The company, he further explained, claims that the mineral water is healthy, pumped directly from a natural spring in Waukesha, Wisconsin, over one hundred miles to the fair.

It was eighty-eight degrees with a cloudless blue sky at 9:00 am, and all four decided to enjoy Hygeia water, preferring an early lunch to breakfast. Unaccustomed to such warm weather and lack of shaded areas, they ducked into the loggia of the ground floor of the Women's Building to quickly drink their water prior to going to the Art Building.

Millie reminded them to hurry, knowing that a crowd would surely gather at the Art Building on the first day of the International Congress of Charities, Correction, and Philanthropy.

Standing in line for admission to the Art Building, Alfred felt a tap on his shoulder.

"Charles, what an unexpected pleasure!" Alfred said, shaking Charles Eliot's hand, a broad smile lighting his face. Having only recently returned from Europe, Alfred had not seen Charles for two months.

"I look forward to reporting on outcomes from our visits once we return after the fair." Alfred mentally scrambled for any memory of the fact that Charles had planned to be in Chicago and came up blank.

Upon noticing Charles with Alfred, Annette broke from her conversation with Millie and Alistair and steered them toward the two men. Smiling and extending her hand, Annette welcomed Charles to the fair, saying that she had not known that he had planned to attend.

"I did not know that I was coming either, Annette, but when I realized that my brother-in-law Francis Peabody, our professor of theology, our *Peabo*, as his students call him, was giving the introductory address to the International Congress today, I knew I needed to be here to support his honorable work in applying Christian ethics to social problems."

Peabo, Charles explained, had radically changed Harvard's compulsory system of religious instruction to a voluntary one, a change applauded by many educators, and one disarming opponents. "He is so quiet and reserved, and so compulsively productive, that it is easy to overlook him," Charles further explained. Annette noticed that Charles, gently scratching the muttonchop on his right cheek with one hand and adjusting his round, wire-rimmed eyeglasses with his other hand, seemed to wilt as he ushered them through the main doors of the building.

"Let's get the best seats, shall we?" Gracious and gentlemanly, Charles gestured for Annette and Millie to take their seats first in a front row, followed by Alfred, Alistair, and himself.

Like school children unsure of their status, Annette and Alfred were edgy, curious if Charles had any reason to attend beyond supporting Peabo. Once they realized he was in Chicago, Millie and Alistair reacted differently, hoping for more time with Charles, keen to understand his thinking, especially about administration and finance of higher education for women. They wondered if they should ask Charles to join them for dinner, and possibly, for time tomorrow to have an update meeting with everyone in Chicago. Progress on topics assigned to Annette, Millie, and Alfred could be reviewed. Millie wanted to learn more about how Charles worked, and Alistair was keen on talking about financial planning. Of all of them, he knew money the best. And Millie knew the details of how things worked.

As attendees filled the great conference hall housing the International Congress of Charities, Correction and Philanthropy, and the din of voices ebbed, Francis G. Peabody was introduced by Charles C. Bonney, president of the World Congress Auxiliary. Bonney, a judge on the Supreme Court of Illinois and a member of the New Jerusalem Church, was the president of all the fair's world congresses and immediately impressed Alfred. Quiet and reserved, Bonney, with his long grey-white beard draping down to his vest, obscuring his starched, high-collared shirt and broad gray necktie, spoke without animation, introducing Peabo with only a brief description.

"Annette, Bonney belongs to my family's church. He is a Swedenborgian." Alfred did not expect Annette to respond, nor did she beyond a courteous nod.

Alfred experienced a sudden, unexpected wave of pride, contrasting dramatically to the growing embarrassment he had been feeling for the past decade about the New Church. Defining himself as Episcopalian in recent years, Alfred now questioned his reasons for leaving behind his Swedenborgian beliefs. He wondered if he simply wished to be more readily accepted within the Back Bay community, by his profession, and at Harvard.

Reasoning that he could not resolve his disquieting thoughts quickly, Alfred turned his attention to the podium, to Peabo, who had now taken center stage. Standing for a moment before beginning, his intense brown eyes peered into his audience. A Unitarian minister deeply embedded in the value of social ethics, Peabo began by noting that the congress was one of self-sacrifice, standing for quiet self-forgetfulness and unassuming devotion.

As Peabo began, Charles excused himself, whispering to Annette that he needed some fresh air.

Annette followed Charles outside the large main doors.

Leaning against the concrete block supporting one of the entrance's massive lions, Charles glanced wearily at Annette as she approached him, asking him if he felt ill. He straightened quickly.

"Do you need anything?" she asked quietly.

"I am fine," Charles retorted briskly. "I simply needed air."

"Yesterday, on our way back to the hotel," Annette remarked, "Alfred and I stopped at a street candy vendor and bought a new treat. It's called Cracker Jacks, caramel-coated popcorn and peanuts. Very tasty." She opened the one-ounce rectangular box, gesturing for him to take a handful.

Feeling trapped, Charles took a handful of Cracker Jacks.

"Truly delicious!" Charles smiled, relaxing his tall frame against the concrete block. He asked for more.

"It's hot, and you probably did not have your usual breakfast. You need sugar. Enjoy them." Annette gave Charles the small box.

Charles confessed that seeing Peabo opened memories well tucked away. Peabo was his brother-in-law and had reminded him of Ellen, Peabo's older sister by eleven years, Charles's first wife. They had four sons, he told Annette, before she died of tuberculosis in October of 1869, only four days after he was named Harvard's twenty-first president.

"She was only thirty-three," he said, looking into the empty box, "when she died."

Charles looked at Annette. She knew she could say nothing to such loss and stood quietly with him as the sugar took its effect and he became himself again. As she had with Alfred, she knew that she could only bear witness.

"I know Peabo well. I am sure he has many more pages to read. We had best rejoin our group before they send out a search party for us."

Ever the administrator, Charles had secured a small conference room in the Arts Building for his planning group to review the status of their work to date. He began his informal meeting with an apology for his poor manners, indicating that he was unable to have food and coffee delivered to their meeting.

"Perhaps," said Millie, a sly grin on her face, "we can enjoy a Pabst Blue Ribbon beer after our meeting. It won the top beer award here at the fair. I'd like to try one!"

"Unusual at midday, but yes, we can taste test the blue-ribbon winner with a late lunch. My treat," said Charles. He had begun to appreciate Millie's contribution to the group, seeing the value of her authentic forthrightness.

The Harvard president pivoted immediately to business.

"Let me describe the progress Elizabeth Agassiz and I have made toward degree-granting for Radcliffe College."

And so, the meeting began. The agenda had been a busy one, with reports on open meetings on the subject of women's education with various groups both within, and beyond, Harvard and the Annex, now called Radcliffe College by Charles. Applauding Elizabeth as a brilliant politician, Charles spoke of her facility to redirect conversations to ensure razor focus on the topic at hand, and to do so with both charm and clarity. Charles reported that in their presentations to both the Harvard Corporation and Board of Overseers, they accomplished their goal — endorsement of degree-granting authority to Radcliffe College. Dangling Harvard's late entrance into the field of women's education, Charles capitalized on pride, suggesting to the board that they had not read the tea leaves well. For her part, Elizabeth provided tables of grades, awards, and other accolades of Annex students, often comparing them to those of Harvard students. Her data was undeniable. The board yielded.

Gathering the additional proponents for degree-granting authority for Radcliffe College, however, had required more than approval of the college's scions. Harvard's, and the Harvard Annex's, alumni were formidable groups, not all committed to the crew's goal. These were people with power and money who had some sway on what their city on the hill should look like.

"What of my father's work, his five-part series in *The Boston Globe*?" Annette asked. She knew that her father's series had now concluded, and that it had been generally well received. Having reviewed his features prior to publication, Annette recognized her father's writing talent, his skill with words, using them as hooks, drawing readers into his view. While it was difficult to measure the direct impact of his series, Annette knew that newspapers were persuasive tools to influence opinion of the powerful opposition.

"Annette, I think that your father will get a Press Club Award for best feature series. His articles may easily sway readers as proponents for women's education." Recognizing talent when he saw it, Charles was effusive regarding Amos's genius with language.

Nodding to Alfred, Charles gestured for the physician to offer his update.

Alfred, clearing his throat, shared his progress report. Proud of his oratory skills and smart demeanor, Alfred loved an audience, including small groups. He and his wife, he reported, had found their trip to Europe fruitful. Grateful that Elizabeth spoke fluent German, Alfred praised German nurses highly, noting that nurse pupils are trained to teach patients anything they can do for themselves, and to help each other in daily care. Teaching self-care was a major tenet of their school, and Alfred noted especially the German belief that independence increases the patient's happiness.

He found this also to be the philosophy at the Royal Infirmary of Edinburgh in Scotland, where ill men helped "care for ailing bairns," a phrase he knew would bring a chuckle from the little room.

"In summary, cleanliness, rigor, adherence to schedules, and regular classes operating under the philosophy of self-care are critical to the successful operation of a school." Alfred, so impressed with the schools he visited, asked if he could take a few more minutes to describe his very different experiences in his own country, most notably at Boston's Lying-In Hospital and San Francisco's County Hospital.

"As clean and orderly as the German and Scottish hospitals were," he reported as he adjusted a cufflink, "that is precisely how filthy and degrading the two hospitals in America were by contrast." Lack of structure, inefficiency, and poor discipline generated chaos, he said, with exhausted pupil nurses and doctors too busy to teach them.

Looking at Annette and Millie, Alfred concluded that a Harvard school of nursing, in addition to promoting a thorough curriculum, must be uncompromising in its principles.

"Alfred, perhaps our first effort in designing a curriculum might be outlining our values and principles," Annette said thoughtfully. Millie nodded affirmatively and added that she loved the principle of patient self-accountability for health. She recalled Lillian Wald's instruction to teach patients to be responsible for themselves, to eliminate behaviors that were hurtful and to embrace healthy behaviors instead.

Alistair, intrigued by Millie's comments, sought examples of healthy versus unhealthy behaviors.

Millie, glancing at Annette, spoke first.

"Excessive alcohol use, cigarette and cigar smoking, gluttony, lack of exercise, and other behaviors. Behaviors that are associated with ill health, even unsafe sexual practices such as having multiple partners." Realizing that the list was too long to detail, Millie asked Annette to provide Alistair examples of healthy behaviors.

Annette stated simply that healthy behaviors were the opposite of what Millie had described as unhealthy behaviors. "Such behaviors are difficult to teach, and even more difficult to embrace," she added.

Checking his pocket watch, Charles thanked Alfred for his update and asked Annette and Millie for an abbreviated summary of their trip to visit Lillian Wald in the Lower East Side. Providing a quick report, Annette indicated that their curriculum focus would be on patients' health maintenance, not simply implementing physicians' disease treatments. Millie added that nursing students would learn to nurse wherever people existed — in homes, hospitals, schools, factories, or elsewhere. In contrast, Millie explained Wald's belief that hospitals house health failures, or, in some cases, injuries from trauma.

Reports complete, Charles then invited Alistair to share his thoughts on the work of the group.

"My thoughts run simple. You will need money for everything you plan on doing. That is where I enter. When you are ready, I can develop a business plan for a Harvard school of nursing, including projected revenue from tuition, construction of an endowment, a five- or ten-year gift-giving campaign, and detailed human and other expenses. I hope to remain privy to your plans, so please keep me in your confidence." Along with his appreciation of Millie, Charles was beginning to realize the financial acumen of Alistair.

"It is now noon. Time for lunch," Charles added with a wink to Millie, "and notwithstanding our caution about alcohol, a Pabst Blue Ribbon beer." Charles picked up his papers, suggesting that they should meet at the Big Tree Restaurant west of the Anthropological Building in thirty minutes.

After a quick lunch and a sip of beer, Charles hailed a single-horse hansom cab and returned to the Grand Passenger Station to board a train back to Boston.

His work in Chicago was finished.

The oxygen returned to the restaurant.

"We shall be leaving soon, and tomorrow we'll be in a conference all day. I suggest we visit the buildings and exhibits we are interested in today," suggested Millie.

They agreed, with Alistair turning to the midway attractions. Alfred headed to the Manufacturing and Liberal Arts Building, and Annette and Millie sauntered toward the Women's Building. Deciding that it was an off-duty afternoon, they planned to meet at the end of the day for a light late-evening dinner at the Philadelphia Cafe just west of the Mines and Mining Building.

"It is imperative you read this," said the Black woman, expressionless, with wide-open brown eyes staring directly at Annette. She asked for a few minutes of her time. Ida B. Wells handed Annette a pamphlet, *Why the Colored American is not in the World's Columbian Exposition*. Annette and Millie had been approaching the Women's Building as Ida rested her hand on Annette's shoulder so she would pause and accept the pamphlet. With neatly coiffed hair atop her head and wearing a high-collared dress with white lace on bodice and sleeves, Ida was a commanding presence. At thirty-one years old, she had become an astute judge of people, realizing in seconds that Annette and Millie were, given their general demeanor, posture, and appearance, perhaps educated women.

Annette and Millie were captivated.

"I am a journalist," Ida said as the three women walked the seven steps to the building's ground floor loggia, facing the midway Plaisance. There, they selected chairs as the sky clouded, with gusty winds and a light rain following.

Intrigued by Ida's seriousness and confidence, Millie asked Ida to kindly tell her more about herself and her work. Although the Civil War had ended twenty-eight years earlier, preceded by President Lincoln's Emancipation Proclamation, rarely had either Annette or Millie seen Black people such as Ida, and never had they interacted with any who looked at them directly on terms that were explicitly equal. Both women were eager to listen.

Ida spoke first of her background and education, beginning with her birth into slavery in Mississippi, her college education, her time as an elementary school teacher, and her work as a journalist. She emphasized her interest in documenting lynching in America. Standing, with a wide sweep of her arm, Ida gestured to the White City, asking them to identify any building devoted to the contributions of Black people in America.

"Despite the urging of Frederick Douglass and other prominent Black people that a separate exhibition hall be built where Black Americans could represent themselves as a unique, contributing racial and ethnic entity," she continued, "their request was denied by the National Directors." She sat as she expressed gratitude to the Republic of Haiti for opening their pavilion in the White City as the single building at the fair representing Americans of African descent.

"It is in the Haiti Pavilion," Ida noted, smiling, "that Frederick Douglass, our august abolitionist and equal rights advocate, acts as leader, representing both the Haitian government and all Blacks during the fair." She described the pamphlet that Annette held as detailing the accomplishments of Black people since the end of the Civil War, including detailed financial achievements and employment gains.

"Protest and pride, this is what the pamphlet represents," Ida said, as she settled into her chair, now comfortable that the two White women had seen her. Millie knew just how important that was. Pointing to the midway Plaisance, Ida described it as a chaotic, unfocused, demeaning array of exhibits and cultures deemed primitive, with disparaging colonial displays of people such as the Dahomeans of West Africa, human beings considered justified trophies of imperialism.

Silent before the implications of the pamphlet and the force of the woman sitting across from them, Annette and Millie had difficulty framing conversation.

Haltingly, Annette asked Ida her thoughts on suffrage.

"I have spent my life as an anti-lynching advocate. I am also a suffragette and equal rights proponent. I abhor stories of Black Sampsons and White Delilahs. Some suffragists are silent on lynching, fighting only for the vote. These core ideas are intermingled; one cannot pick and choose among them."

Remaining on the loggia, the three women sat in silence. Then, with perfect phrasing, Ida returned Millie's question. "Kindly," Ida said with a little smile, "tell me more about yourselves and what it is that you do."

They gave brief summaries of their education but spent more time talking about their current involvement in efforts to ensure educational opportunities for women and training of nurses.

Then, on impulse, Annette asked the question: "Would you consider being a guest speaker at the Harvard Annex on the topics of equal rights, anti-lynching, and suffrage?"

She was beginning to understand just how radically, and quickly, her world was changing. If she and her peers were to advocate for women's education, then ideas broader than simply gender required exploration. Race, not only gender, was critically important to consider. She feared she and Millie might be White Delilahs in the White City. If so, she knew this whiteness would not do.

Ida agreed to visit the Annex, adding that oppression might be the most poignant topic of interest, a word best summarizing the breadth of their conversation. While attempting to focus on Ida's comments, Annette invariably thought of the ascetic training of pupil nurses. Yes, oppression indeed.

Serving as Ida's surrogates, Annette and Millie agreed to distribute a handful of her pamphlets as they strolled through the exhibits at the Women's Building. After saying their goodbyes, Annette and Millie walked slowly on the steps of the grand landing of the center terrace past the John Philip Sousa band playing "The Stars and Stripes Forever." Immediately following the band, a poet read Katharine Lee Bates's "America the Beautiful," to hearty cheers of spectators.

In their silence, Millie reflected on the fact that Americans were such a complex, confused people. For her part, Annette realized that the Civil War had not yet ended. They now heard the march and the poem in ways far different than those surrounding them.

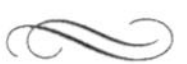

Entering the Women's Building from the west portico, Annette and Millie checked their light shawls with a clerk at the sales room, picked up a slim guidebook, and walked slowly into the main rotunda. A decorated skylight and rows of clerestory windows brilliantly lit the large interior central rotunda, a charming sensory effect interrupted only by the echoing created by their heeled Balmoral boots as they struck the floor.

They explored the art tastefully displayed in the exhibit stands in the gallery, amazed that such delicate work had been organized in such a short period. The knowledge that the building itself, as was true with other buildings in the White City, was temporary only for the duration of the fair both deeply impressed and unsettled them. The White City announced that America was the world's new lead republic, signifying freedom, success, and liberty. Virtue abounded. Yet there was Ida herself, testament that what was true for some was not true for all.

Entering the library off the west side of the gallery, Annette and Millie hungrily surveyed multiple book collections by female writers from all over the country, as well as books by foreign women writers. Sitting in comfortable chairs designed to provide a cozy atmosphere conducive for reading, they combed through the collection of one hundred books written by Massachusetts women between the years 1612 and 1893.

Looking up briefly from a book, Annette was surprised to see Claire Williams, president of the Boston regional chapter of the General Federation of Women's Clubs, enter the library with Frances Willard, whom she had not seen since the two met in Boston at Claire's home. Annette recalled what the president of the Women's Christian Temperance Union had said to her: "Prohibition of alcohol and birth control are needed at the same time. *Now!*" Annette stood, happy to see this social activist again.

"How wonderful to see you!" Annette exclaimed, giving Claire a quick hug and Frances a handshake, and reintroducing Millie to them. Both women were at the fair representing their organizations. Gathering their belongings, Annette and Millie walked with Claire and Frances up to the Garden Café on the third floor at the south end. There, they enjoyed tall glasses of sweetened iced green tea. After a quick review of local club happenings, Claire asked Frances if she had seen the pastel drawing by Henrietta Briggs-Wall displayed in the gallery.

"Yes, I have seen it. In fact, I worked with Henrietta from her very conception of the drawing." Frances explained that the drawing, which superficially portrayed her in a very unflattering light, placed her in the center with four men surrounding her. One represented a mentally disabled man, another a convict, a third a madman, and the fourth a Native American.

"The message, you see, is that neither American women nor undesirable classes of men had been granted equal voting rights." Frances noted that Henrietta believed the drawing shocking to many viewers, but shock, she had claimed, aroused some people to a sense of injustice and degradation regarding women in America. Frances reminded them that they could purchase postcards of the drawing, *American Woman and her Political Peers*, at the sales room on the west side of the rotunda, ground floor.

"These postcards have also been published internationally," Frances added.

Recovering as best she could from the realization that Willard, socially alert, was nevertheless oblivious to the fact that she herself was as blindly dismissive of others as those who denied women the vote, Millie turned the conversation to Ida Wells. Millie briefly summarized their conversation on the loggia, handing Frances a copy of Wells's pamphlet.

"Ida and I agree on equal rights for women. However, we have been at odds over her anti-lynching campaign. The Women's Christian Temperance Union is primarily involved in alcoholic temperance and suffrage for women, while Ida, additionally, is deeply devoted to anti-lynching. She thinks me a coward because I have not publicly denounced lynching."

Frances hesitated for a moment, as if seriously considering her next words.

"In October, 1890, I was quoted in the *New York Voice* as having said that the colored race multiplies like the locusts of Egypt, that the grog-shop is the center of power, that plantation Negros unable to read nor write should not be entrusted with the ballot. I never, however, condoned lynching. Ida and I agree that lawlessness cannot be tolerated in our country."

Frances sipped her drink. Annette and Millie, in stunned silence, waited to see if anything further was forthcoming.

"We remain a divided country," Frances added, "irrespective of Civil War outcomes." She thanked her companions for their lively discussions, and then departed.

Claire, Annette, and Millie looked at each other and, without speaking a word, ordered tall glasses of Regent's punch, cold tea flavored with pineapple, orange, and dark Jamaican rum.

And, after the first, each enjoyed second drinks. Concerning Frances and her views, they tacitly decided that silence was best if, for no other reason, they did not know where to begin with hatred running so deep.

Prior to departing for a light dinner with the rest of their group, Annette asked Claire about Ellen, knowing that she had not been feeling well at their last visit.

"Annette, you may wish to visit your aunt when you return. She is a very proud woman, and I fear she is keeping her illness a secret from her family. Weak with troublesome coughing and poor sleep, Ellen leaves her home infrequently and seems to be avoiding medical care. She truly loves you. Perhaps you may get a better sense of her health."

Annette assured Claire that she would surely see Ellen when back in Cambridge over the upcoming weekend.

Each day, Annette thought, complexities grew, almost as quickly as women's restlessness.

On route to the Philadelphia Café in the Mines and Mining Building, Annette and Millie found Alistair with a new friend, introduced as David Furst, on the walkway adjoining the wooded aisle with the targeted building. After a light dinner, all agreed to rejoin in the morning for a brisk walk to the Arts Building to attend the Section III sessions on hospitals, dispensaries, and nursing.

A sweltering hot sun accompanied Annette, Millie, Alfred, and Alistair as they walked, undaunted, toward the Art Institute. Glancing at the majestic lions as they climbed the two short flights of steps on the Michigan Avenue entrance of the building, they eagerly entered the atrium, pleased for the cool, shady space.

In a large meeting room in the second-floor eastern annex, attendees of the Section III session — *Hospital Care of the Sick, Training of Nurses, Dispensary Work, and First Aid to the Injured* — were taking their seats. John S. Billings, chairman of the Congress, arranged his papers at the podium. Meticulously groomed, with hair center-parted and accented by a long whitish-gray goatee mustache and chin beard, Billings commanded attention. A renowned battlefield surgeon during the Civil War, Billings had designed and supervised the construction of the Johns Hopkins Hospital in Maryland, including plans for a four-year medical school and related health research.

Calling the general session meeting to order at 10 am on June 14th, Billings struck the sound block with his gavel. This was a part of the fair that Annette anticipated since Charlotte Macleod had told her about it at Waltham.

"As we indicated in the January 28, 1893, issue of *The Hospital*," he began, "this Congress will have fifteen subjects for special consideration. Miss Isabel A. Hampton, superintendent of the Training School for Nurses of the Johns Hopkins Hospital, has been appointed president of the session related to the training of nurses." After relaying details related to sectional sessions, Billings set the tone for the Congress in his address, entitled *The Relations of Hospitals to Public Health.*

Alfred, a particularist, had admired Billings's work as a statistician, librarian, hospital designer, and educator. He well knew Billings's reorganization of the Marine Hospital Fund following the Civil War and appreciated the work conducted by the Marine Hospital in Boston, the oldest hospital in Massachusetts. While on rotation at the Lying-In Hospital in Boston in 1883, Alfred was appalled at both the septic environment and the abysmal disarray of patient records. Following Billings's principles of census reporting used in the tabulation of statistics for the US census in 1880 and 1890, Alfred had designed a system of patient census that identified each patient, dates of hospitalization, and diagnosis. From Billings's indexing system of medical periodicals to his establishment of the surgeon general's library, Alfred was inspired by Billings, whom he considered a multitalented medical icon.

At the edge of his seat, Alfred attended to Billings's address to the exclusion of any audience whispers and chair scraping in the conference room. Although Billings's voice was somewhat high-pitched and, judging by the reactions of Millie and Alistair, irritating, Alfred found his message spot-on, congruent with Waltham Hospital's mission and values. Emphasizing that hospitals established after the Civil War were critical for the proper and complete training of physicians, surgeons, and nurses, Billings posed the question of whether a network of hospitals should be established under national control, to be supplied from national funds, to be free to everyone, similar to the nationalization of health proposal offered by Havelock Ellis the previous year. Billings affirmed that teaching hospitals provide the skilled doctors and nurses needed by patients in their homes and communities, with practitioners capable of promoting the public's health and safety.

Fascinated by Billings's statement that curious questions of jurisdiction might arise if standards for medical and nursing education were regulated by the state, Alfred recalled Charlotte Macleod's concern that current nurse leaders were demanding strict regulation of nursing by state boards. Here to listen and understand national perspectives regarding hospitals and nursing education, Alfred focused especially on Billings's caution on overregulation.

Billings's address ended with a rousing applause. The audience, particularly Alfred, had been captivated by his insightful ideas coupling hospitals to education and public health. His nuanced comments on possible state regulation of educational standards stimulated interest among attendees, with many crowding the podium to speak with him after his session. While not discourteous, Billings brusquely gestured his goodbyes to his audience, and exited the conference room. Another important man in a hurry, Alfred thought. After a brief intermission, the conference resumed, with papers presented by Isabel A. Hampton and Lavinia Dock.

Annette and Millie were eager for the presentation on the *Educational Standards for Nurses*, to be given by Hampton. Annette recollected Alfred's previous description of Hampton, recalling that physician William Osler described her as an animated Greek statue. Annette was fascinated by accounts of Hampton's quiet demeanor, strong work ethic, and focused determination to transform nursing from the public's perception of drunken Sairy Gamp to that of a trained professional. Charlotte Macleod had also been complimentary of Hampton, a rare exception to the Waltham nursing superintendent's typical assessment of current nurse leaders. What would Isabel look like? How would she sound?

Unlike Annette, Millie was more interested in Hampton's nursing textbook. Through Annette, Millie had obtained a copy of the book—a doorstop, she thought—with twenty-eight chapters and over five hundred pages. While she had not yet had time to complete it, she had devoured chapter one in just two days, noting nursing's radically different curriculum plan from her own in the classics. Hampton described a twenty-four-month hospital training, divided into nine rotations mirroring hospital departments. Medical, surgical, and gynecological rotations involved five months' time each, with children, operating room, private wards, special duty, dispensary, and cooking school each spanning one- to two-month experiences. Also suggesting library holdings and detailed topics for weekly lectures and demonstrations, Hampton recommended that examinations of first-year content must be passed in order to progress to the second year. Unlike her own academic year, Millie soon realized that pupil nurses would have eight months of lectures and bedside care delivery during winter months, followed by four months of only practical nursing in the summer. Both physicians and the nursing superintendent comprised the training program faculty. All the time, it seemed, everybody was on duty.

With dark-brown hair arranged in an unruly bun, Hampton began her presentation humbly, expressing her topic — educational standards for nurses — as very important and complex, since it dealt with the problems of health and disease, of life and death. Speaking softly and scanning her audience carefully, Hampton established that modern nursing was routinely offered in schools established by hospitals. Upon graduation, trained nurses were employed in private duty, district nursing, or, occasionally, missionary nursing. She described the exceptional qualifications required for trained nursing, including mental, moral, and physical strength, in addition to infinite tact.

Claiming that a school of nursing is established to provide the sponsoring hospital with a reliable corps of nurses, Hampton frowned — physically while reading, Annette noticed — on pupil nurses participating in care of families in their homes, saying that doing so secures income for the hospital at the expense of students' education. Most importantly, she urged that schools conduct a uniform system of instruction in programs lengthened to three years with eight hours daily of practical work. Domestic science, or home education, stressed Hampton, was a critical prerequisite to nurse training, since nurses are the stewards of hospital property and thus, ultimately, hospital finances.

Hampton, seeming earnest and sincere to Annette, concluded her presentation by stating, in aphorism, that "the head, the heart, and the hand" of a true nurse must work in harmony on behalf of patients. It was quite the ending.

Annette, Millie, Alfred, and Alistair took solace in the uniformity of their silence, a validation of their contrary opinions from those of the audience, now clapping vigorously.

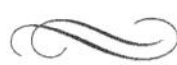

As Lavinia Dock walked to the podium to give her address on the relationship between training schools and hospitals, Annette and Millie watched her stately stride, recalling their brief, testy exchange at Claire's Boston home earlier that year.

"Shall we wave at her," Millie giggled to Annette, "and yell out to the dowager that the non-nurses are here, barbarians at the gate, civilization lost?"

"Perhaps not just yet," Annette replied. She knew that women of Lavinia's class were dangerous, and she intuitively felt that Dock would resist, even work to ruin, everything she was working to accomplish.

Dock began with a review of the history of nurses' training since the Civil War, noting especially the relationship between sponsoring hospitals and training schools for nurses, the singular question being which came first: the hospital or the school? Indicating that a nursing school comes properly "under the command of the medical profession," specifically relative to the direct care of the sick, she inferred that nursing schools were essential equipment for hospitals.

"Here, indeed," Lavinia noted with a little sniff, "the command is absolute." Expanding on what she clearly considered a foundational truth, she added, again, with a sniff, that the nurse must proudly provide perfect service "faithfully, fully, and at all hours" in a hospital.

Obedience to orders was the dominant characteristic of the new system of nursing, enabling nursing to flourish as a profession. Regarding the material prosperity of hospitals, she proposed that such success would be due to the work of the training school, resulting in improved outcomes, less infection, and quicker recoveries. The costs associated with training schools are acceptable, she offered, since schools are flexible instruments, less expensive than retaining a graduate nurse staff. Additionally, the discipline and strict subordination of the school to the hospital make the amount of work performed by pupil nurses possible, quite contrary to that of a paid staff.

As the presentation concluded, Annette noticed that Millie was literally sitting on her hands.

"I need to understand what these women are promoting. I also need a drink!" said Alistair, as they left the conference hall following Dock's address, rejoining the lions on the steps of the Art Institute.

Settling for glasses of Hygeia Waukesha water sold at a food cart, the crew walked to the loggia of the Women's Building, seeking comfort in shade, away from nurses gathering for breaks outside the Art Institute.

Realizing they had much to consider, they sat in uncharacteristic silence, knowing that they were to attend additional presentations shortly. Upon return to the conference room, to see if any activity remained that was not on the program, they were surprised to see Isabel Hampton again at the podium.

Thanking the audience for allowing her to make an announcement, Hampton reported that several nursing superintendents at the conference had requested the establishment of an Association of Superintendents of Training Schools. Seeking approval, she asked for a show of hands from those in agreement with the idea. Her request was quickly followed by the thunder of clapping hands.

"Such a cordial response," she said to the audience, clearly pleased yet surprised by the overwhelmingly positive feedback. She then gestured to K. L. Lett, superintendent of St. Luke's Hospital in Chicago, who extended an invitation to several superintendents to join her in her sitting room the following day upon completion of all presentations to discuss detailed next steps.

Following this brief announcement, the participants left the room. Annette, Millie, Alfred, and Alistair found themselves again by the lions.

Annette and Millie, not invited to Lett's private meeting in her sitting room, were frustrated. Annette's experiences over the last year had led them to understand that important decisions were made in such closed rooms.

"I will ask if I can attend," said Alfred. He noted that he could serve as Charlotte Macleod's designee.

"Alfred," laughed Alistair, "you represent the very people they *don't want to attend!*"

"Frankly," he continued, "it would be easier for me to attend than you. Women are generally not put off by me."

In a withering tone they had come to know, Millie reminded both men that, while women still did not vote in America, they were learning the power of organizing. Working up steam, Millie noted that the General Federation of Women's Clubs, the Women's Christian Temperance Union, even the National American Woman Suffrage Association, knew that results are best achieved through organizational structure, designing strategies to effect true change. Paternalism, she continued, was not welcome, neither from the good doctor nor the charming financier.

Annette, smiling, agreed with Millie, adding that nursing superintendents must concur on their goals before inviting anyone, whether men or women, to support their mission.

The two men looked at the ground, appearing to have suddenly taken an interest in their shoes.

The next day, Thursday, June 15th, after sessions of the nursing subsection closed, Hampton, true to her promise, invited superintendents of training schools to remain to discuss the possibility of establishing an organization for nursing superintendents.

Annette understood, but was enraged nonetheless. Millie, prior to leaving the room, quickly surveyed the eighteen women who remained. She noted that Miss C. E. M. Somerville, from Lawrence General Hospital in Lawrence, Massachusetts, was present in the room. Somerville had presented the previous day on district nursing in America, calling it a distinct branch, one dependent on hospital-trained nurses to care for the sick poor in their homes, those unable to pay for either private-duty nurses or hospital care. Somerville, a disciple of Amy Hughes, superintendent of the Metropolitan and National Nursing Association, London, recognized the values of both hospital sick training and home training. The "Met," as Hughes identified the British association, was founded in 1874 to raise the standards of care in district nursing. Hughes had presented the previous day as well, and both women's presentations were warmly received, with vivid descriptions of the responsibilities of district nurses, considered infinitely greater than those of one working in a hospital with the doctors to turn to, according to Hughes.

"We will befriend Somerville, a Massachusetts colleague," declared Millie, speaking to Annette and Alfred.

As the women filed out of the room and headed towards Lett's parlor, Millie approached Somerville, asking if she and Annette could speak with her the next morning at breakfast.

"Of course. It will be lovely to hear your Boston accents after so many hours of foreign speakers," Somerville said playfully, with a wink to Hughes.

The day behind them, the crew returned to the lions, milled about, and left.

"Livestock Pavilion?" asked Alistair. It was 7:30 am on Friday, June 16th, and the sun was already blazing. Millie raised her eyebrows at Alistair, who knew that she had arranged a breakfast meeting with Miss Somerville at the French bakery east of the Livestock Pavilion to learn results of the superintendents' discussion the day before. Was Alistair suggesting that there were more cows to see in addition to those at lecterns yesterday? They both burst out laughing together.

Somerville had saved a table for them at the bakery and was now riffling through her papers. A short, well-rounded older woman, she wore a light blue day dress and carried a white lacy portable parasol and a leather briefcase. With gray-white hair and a broad smile, she was warm and welcoming.

Millie introduced Annette, Alfred, and Alistair to Somerville, who ordered croissants, scones, and dark roast French coffee for everyone.

Down to business, Somerville summarized the meeting at Lett's parlor. The eighteen superintendents had unanimously celebrated the many advantages of forming an association. They had formed a temporary organization with Anna L. Alston, superintendent of Mount Sinai Training School in New York, as chairman. A committee of eight superintendents framed draft resolutions to be voted on that very day. Somerville paused, taking a sip of coffee.

"This is a marvelous day for nursing!" she added spontaneously, with great enthusiasm.

"What are the draft resolutions?" asked Annette, pulling the balloon back to earth. Anxious to know details, she was working hard to seem casual. Pen in hand, she looked directly at Somerville.

"Dear, our recommendations are simple. We wish to be known as the American Society of Superintendents of Training Schools for Nurses in the United States and Canada. The objectives of our society will be to promote fellowship of members, to establish and maintain a universal standard of training, and to further the best interests of the nursing profession."

Apologizing for taking time to take a substantial bite of her scone, Miss Somerville again paused. After finishing her coffee, she added that a very important aspect of the society would be the qualifications of members. She explained that members must be superintendents of recognized general hospitals giving no less than two years course of instruction. She recalled a lively discussion about a fixed, standard, uniform curriculum, provided in hospitals offering specific services with a minimum number of beds. Like Rome, she noted, a standard curriculum would not be determined in a day, but rather over time. At their first annual meeting, the superintendents planned to write their constitution and elect officers. That meeting was to be held in New York City, in January, the following year.

"Nurse training will be provided in hospitals?" asked Alistair.

"Where else, dear, can nurse training occur?" Realizing that Alistair was a banker ignorant of patient care, she was patient with his questions.

"Who teaches nursing in hospitals?" Alistair continued. He had, by now, shifted to his most sincere look, the eager student desirous of knowledge.

"As you can imagine, the doctors are the most knowledgeable. They will instruct when patient care allows. The superintendents also teach."

"Miss Somerville," Annette asked as Somerville polished off the rest of her croissant, "what does the patient first principle mean to you?" She thought it wise to interrupt Alistair's line of seemingly innocent yet deliberatively provocative questions.

"Hospitals exist for sick patients. Doctors admit patients, and pupil nurses care for them, carrying out doctors' orders. Patients will always come first; teaching is secondary. Classes can be rescheduled."

Sensing that her explanation was insufficient, Somerville further explained that pupil nurses obey doctors' orders, maintain absolute cleanliness according to sanitary principles, prevent infection, and remain on duty all day, every day. She was now eyeing Alistair's croissant.

"Do you think that nursing requires college instruction?" Alistair asked as he placed his croissant in front of her, appalled that she considered hospital training a form of education and wagering that, the more he fed her, the more she would reveal herself.

"I support college education for women, but certainly *not for nursing*. How can a woman learn to nurse in a classroom?" She wrapped the croissant in a napkin and slipped it into her briefcase. Suspecting that she was among wolves and no longer smiling, Somerville said her goodbyes, leaving them to ponder differences in the words *training* and *education*.

Millie turned to Annette and, with a theatrical sigh, reported that befriending the Croissant General, as she would now be forever called by the crew, was not one of her stellar ideas.

Alistair broke the silence after Somerville bustled away.

"Lincoln issued his Emancipation Proclamation thirty years ago. Apparently, he did not free pupil nurses from the slavery of hospitals."

"How can these women think this is right?" Alistair asked, looking to Alfred for a response.

Alfred had been quiet through Somerville's descriptions of the previous evening's events. Alistair's stare tore through Alfred. Realizing that he must respond, Alfred finally spoke.

"I am befuddled, and my world seems topsy-turvy." It seemed the most honest answer. Alfred said that he needed time to understand everything Somerville shared, particularly in relation to Waltham Training School. Slumped in his chair, Alfred remained quiet. His thoughts were dark, tainted with self-anger and embarrassment. Education had always been critically important to him, and he wondered why on earth, knowing what he now knew, he had designed a nursing school built to meet the needs of a hospital. However unwitting, had he begun a nursing school merely to serve the needs of doctors?

In feelings bordering on horror, Alfred saw that his Waltham program improved patients' outcomes, but also provided him an easier lifestyle while insuring income for the hospital. All of this, he now realized, was at the expense of the pupil nurse, deceived to think that her enforced obedience, poor education, and excessive on-duty hours were privileges of engagement with doctors and patients.

When he finally spoke, it was clear to Annette and Millie that Alfred was thinking aloud.

"When we first gathered, you will recall Charles warning us that many snakes in the grass might hinder our efforts to establish a Harvard school of nursing. Such snakes exist. It appears that I may be among them."

Alfred continued, noting that, since the Civil War, hospitals had flourished, but only when buttressed by training schools for nurses. Capitalism had resulted in hospitals becoming synonymous with sick care. Doctors, over forty years ago, established the American Medical Association to secure their interests and to promote the science and art of medicine. But that, it now seemed, was at a great expense. In this light, the architects, anthropologists, artists, electricians, engineers, horticulturalists, and miners featured at the fair itself were envisioning a future for a limited few. Even Charles's aim to Harvardize American education would come at a cost to those who would not fit into his imagined future. Alfred was beginning to see the entire landscape and sat in silence.

Annette finally spoke. "What you are now realizing, Alfred, is that all the noble sentiments on earth are worth little if they exist only in the White City. It may just be that you were, whether you knew it or not, an architect. You didn't know that you would find yourself among the Dahomeans."

Annette, Millie, and Alfred walked in silence back to the Columbian Central Hotel and prepared for their departure the next day. As Annette spoke, Alistair knew, more profoundly than ever, that he was among the Others. He left to find David and be among his own.

Once back in Cambridge, Annette visited her Aunt Ellen, just as Claire had suggested in Chicago. Claire had been correct. Ellen was seriously ill.

Ellen's fatigue was now chronic, her appetite poor. Daytime was fraught with frequent shortness of breath and chest pain exacerbated by coughing. She filled her linen handkerchiefs with blood, quickly folded them, and tucked them into her sleeves. Sleep eluded her, compounded by night sweats. She stripped the pillowcases and scrubbed them back to white herself along with the handkerchiefs. Occasionally, her heart raced, a sensation accompanied by a feeling that it would leap from her chest. When this onset occurred in the presence of others, Ellen became more and more proficient at finding a chair while laughing that the conversation was simply overwhelming. But, in time, the deception had failed, and she had withdrawn from the society she so loved.

"Annette, you are a breath of fresh air!" exclaimed Ellen as she stretched out her arms to encircle her niece.

Propped up by pillows and thick comforters, Ellen was now essentially confined to bed, exhaustion overwhelming her.

"I fear that I can no longer enjoy a cigarette with you in the backyard." Laughing, she became quiet for a moment. "So much excitement," she said. Yet, even among the pillows, Ellen remained the vibrant, intense hero that Annette so admired.

"And now to business."

Ellen told Annette that she had tuberculosis, although she hadn't any recollection of being among anyone with the disease.

"Perhaps," she said, winking at Annette, "one of the fine ladies in our regional Federation Club has shared it with me."

"How do you get along in your day? Can Uncle Stubby help you? Who prepares your meals?" Annette had many questions. Ellen's answers were surprising.

"Stubby helps me a great deal, especially in the morning and at bedtime. He has always been there for me."

"But your mother has saved me. She comes over almost every day, bringing newspapers, books, treats, and anything that she thinks will fill my time. She has even tried to teach me to knit! Can you imagine that?" Ellen pointed to a basket of brightly colored wool on a stand by her bedside woven into delightfully irregular patterns, testament to Caroline's efforts.

"Your mother is different these days. She seems to be open to new ideas, sometimes even asking about women's voting and college education. I think you have changed her over time. And, whatever you, Charles, and Alfred are doing together fascinates her. In fact, I think she may be jealous of your father's involvement through his newspaper articles." Hopeful that she was beginning to view the world beyond the confines of her kitchen, they were heartened as they considered the new Caroline stepping, at last, into the sun.

"Ellen, may I ask Alfred to examine you? He is an expert in tuberculosis and has treated many patients at the Waltham Hospital."

During Annette's visit to Waltham Hospital months earlier, Alfred had indicated that Robert Koch, a German scientist, had discovered a decade ago that pulmonary tuberculosis was an infection caused by the tubercle bacillus. Describing his treatment of tuberculosis with the Carasso method, Alfred had indicated that inhalation of peppermint vapors, or essence of Mentha, serves as a general disinfectant and appetite enhancer. While there was still no definitive cure, patients oftentimes improved using the Carasso method.

Ellen welcomed any treatment that Alfred thought appropriate.

Annette adjusted Ellen's pillows and placed her knitting on a stand next to fresh flowers. Kissing her cheek gently, Annette bid Ellen goodbye.

After examining Ellen later in the week, Alfred suggested that she be treated at Waltham Hospital, with the Carasso method, fresh air, and appetizing meals. Ellen agreed that she would begin her hospital stay.

Following the examination, Alfred told Annette that, since Ellen was an incipient case, hospitalization was a treatment option for her. If she were a terminal case, then Alfred would have recommended a trendle waterbed and supportive care at home. In Massachusetts, he continued, physicians were beginning to see the value of sanitoria for management of early-stage cases.

Alfred noted that the state had begun to plan for a state hospital, a tuberculosis sanitorium, possibly located in Rutland, about sixty miles from Boston. Given that consumption remained the leading cause of death in adults, he explained that medical students see fewer patients with other illnesses since less beds are available.

"This limits their clinical education," he concluded. "We must find ways to manage tuberculosis patients other than in our general hospitals. I'll keep you informed of our progress toward that goal." Alfred helped Ellen settle into a lounge chair with footrest on Waltham Hospital's wide porch, adjusting her pillows for comfort.

Kissing her cheek gently, Annette bid Ellen goodbye, as Caroline moved her bedside stand closer to her chair.

"I'll be back soon," promised Caroline. "I really want to understand the political issues surrounding women's education." As Caroline turned her back, Ellen and Annette shared a smile, with Ellen mimicking a long drag on an imaginary cigarette.

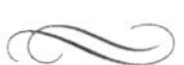

"Alfred, you are not yourself. Since you returned from Chicago, you are edgy and short-tempered. Do you wish to talk?" His wife, Elizabeth, put down her book, leaned forward in her parlor chair, and took Alfred's hands in her own.

"Elizabeth, I fear I have made a terrible error in judgement," replied Alfred, his voice low, almost inaudible. "And no amount of clever talk will erase that."

Elizabeth waited. Recognizing his discomfort, she simply continued to hold his hand.

In March of 1885, Alfred reminisced, he and four physician friends—Edward R. Cutler, J. W. Willis, C. J. McCormick, and W. F. Jarvis—had published a circular in the *Waltham Free Press* announcing the opening of the Waltham Training School for Nurses. But now, looking back from the vantage point he had seen in Chicago, he wondered why he had been so eager to establish the school. He now realized that he wished to alleviate the burden on himself and other doctors and to help patients improve. While he thought of nursing as a field giving women paying jobs, he also admitted that he saw it as a field not competing with men, specifically, doctors.

"Elizabeth, home calls were exhausting me. Hospitals, especially those with training schools, offered relief, both for me and for patients. Other than giving women future jobs in private duty, I did not think of women as students in any way. What type of education do they deserve? Must they live under enforced rule, without the joys of college education? They are taught to obey rather than to seek knowledge. Trained to be silent rather than inquisitive."

Alfred had begun to pace.

"I have been selfish." He remained silent for a few moments.

"But this does not need to continue," he said, raising his head, his voice surer than previously.

"What are your options?" Elizabeth prodded.

"Two options, Elizabeth. Make no change, or transition to a college program at Harvard, ceasing admissions to the Waltham training school once the degree program opens." To Elizabeth, Alfred seemed relieved to have spoken aloud.

He continued, noting that if a Harvard four-year nursing degree program began in fall, 1900, then the three-year Waltham program would admit its last class that same year. This sequence, he computed, would allow Waltham's last graduation to be in 1903, with Harvard's first graduation to be in 1904. Such a planned sequence would prevent any gap in the graduation of nurses for the community.

"What are your thoughts, Elizabeth?" Alfred stopped pacing, looking directly at his wife.

He knew that she had spoken to many of Harvard's faculty, as well as medical and dental school alumni, concerning the award of degree-granting authority to the Annex. Elizabeth described their reactions when faced with objective, dispassionate information on the subject.

"In these meetings, most agree that a woman must have the same right to college education as a man. But, remember, I only spoke of the Annex, not to the idea of establishing a school of nursing at Harvard." Elizabeth predicted that getting consensus for a school of nursing at Harvard might be far trickier, especially with doctors privately worried about possible competition. She suggested that his first step might be to speak with his physician colleagues at Waltham Hospital.

"Encourage them," Elizabeth counselled, "to predict possible disadvantages to *them* if the training school were to close. What advantages, if any, might they *gain* with a Harvard school of nursing? They must see more wins than losses. Appeal to ego and finances. If your Waltham Hospital colleagues ultimately design such a transition plan as you describe, then you have a powerful political ally." Alfred agreed with Elizabeth, recognizing that her political acumen stemmed both from education and years of navigating her father through murky situations as Harvard's twentieth president.

Elizabeth offered to host a dinner party for the key founding physicians of the Waltham Hospital Training School for Nurses. Charles Eliot; Elizabeth Agassiz; Amos Fiske and his wife,

Caroline; Annette; Alistair; and Millie would also be invited. A capable, charismatic organizer, Elizabeth arranged a dinner in ten days' time, accented with piano music and singing by Marguerite, Annette's sister.

As Elizabeth planned her dinner party over the next few days, Alfred sought advice from his friend and colleague, Edward Cutler, one of Waltham's most beloved doctors and an advocate of the training school. Meeting on a hot, sunny day as they sat in rocking chairs on his sheltered front porch, Cutler sipped his hot coffee, noting that he was forever cold in his old age. Stout, with suspenders crisscrossed in the back, snugly retaining his wide girth in his dark-brown pants, he presided confidently on his porch. Even as he rocked with his eyes somewhat closed, Cutler was keenly aware of, and interested in, Alfred's proposal.

When Alfred finished, Cutler's eyes snapped open. Gone was the old fellow. Present was the adventurous colleague.

"Say no more, Alfred. We may have been unwittingly cruel in our original design of the training school, benefiting enormously by the work of pupil nurses. Without malice intent, we became hospital capitalists, enjoying a more peaceful lifestyle due to the work of pupils. But I agree with you. It is time for change. We must be on the better side of history regarding women's education."

Cutler agreed to lead the discussion at Elizabeth's upcoming dinner party. As he puffed his cigar and sipped his strong hot coffee, he promised not to let Alfred down.

Charlotte Macleod and her young friend, Susan Patterson, mounted the two-horse hansom cab outside the Waltham Training School for Nurses, on route to a meeting at Fay House in Cambridge.

Both women were honored to be invited to the Harvard Annex. Allowing Charlotte an off-duty day to plan essentials for a nursing baccalaureate-level program, Alfred requested that she review Waltham's current admission criteria as well as those of other training programs.

Regarding the Waltham program, Alfred's request was an easy one for Charlotte.

For comparison to criteria used by other programs, however, Charlotte sought help from Susan, her young friend who had graduated in 1891 from the Newark City Hospital Training School for Nurses in New Jersey. When her father died shortly after her graduation, Susan returned to Waltham to live with her mother, becoming a private-duty nurse. Charlotte, eleven years Susan's senior, became her advisor and friend after they met at a local Episcopal Church community event.

Grateful and loyal to Charlotte for her guidance, Susan was eager to describe her training program, especially her rotations to clinical services. Tall, thin, with short, cropped black hair, deep-set brown eyes, and plainly dressed, Susan was quite different in appearance from both Annette and Millie but similar in her confidence. Like them, she knew where she stood in the world.

When Susan arrived at Faye House, Annette shook her hand and thanked her for her willingness to share her expertise with the group. After introducing herself, Susan chose a place at the circular conference table, large enough to accommodate ten people comfortably.

Millie spread her papers on the table, then, predictably, galvanized the group to action, rolling a large portable blackboard into the drawing parlor serving as their conference center. She asked Charlotte to describe the basis of admission to the Waltham School.

"Let's start," Millie said, chalk in hand. Charlotte, unsure whether to stand or remain seated, looked to Alfred, her cheeks gradually reddening as she spoke. Alfred nodded, encouraging her to begin. She remained seated, knowing that she could see everyone at the table clearly.

"When Waltham moved from a farming village to a factory city," said Charlotte, with confidence in her voice, "families' care needs became greater, friendly visiting by neighbors faded, and doctors couldn't find enough nurses for private-duty care." Charlotte recalled that as the city grew, along with increased industrial injuries and infectious diseases, Alfred called for the establishment of both a hospital and a nurses' training school. Rather than teaching family members to care for ill patients at home, Alfred, according to Charlotte, believed that young women could be trained as doctors' nursing assistants, thus freeing doctors for other tasks. Such assistants, he believed, could give valuable care to patients as well as relief for busy country doctors.

"Beginning on April 17th, 1885, Dr. Edward Cutler started lecturing to six students every Monday afternoon in the parlor of Mary Piper's boarding house on Main Street. Mary Hacket was brought on as superintendent after the first year, when the future of the school seemed fairly well assured." Charlotte added that the school itself was officially incorporated on February 24th,1888, almost three years after its establishment.

"I am reticent to tell you the admission criteria for the Waltham School," Charlotte said, a worried expression on her face, fearing that the group might think her school lax.

She recalled that, eight years ago, a small handful of people started both the school and hospital for a variety of reasons. At that time, she explained, the old bias against nurses as dissolute midwives prevailed. Parents, she claimed, looked askance at nursing, believing mandatory nursing service in almshouses or prisons was frequently meted out as punishment for criminal behavior.

"The school's founders had to actively push back against this prejudice," Charlotte claimed, "as they started nurses' training without any precedents to guide them, and with no available funding. The school was needed. It was a new undertaking. In 1885, it began, informally."

Admission criteria, according to Charlotte, evolved over time. To have a school, she noted, young women needed to be admitted. Without students, the experiment of a training school could not be undertaken. If young women could be persuaded to enter the program, then criteria could be discerned over time for what kind of women they must be.

"So, you see, in the beginning, there were no entrance requirements," Charlotte explained.

She recalled that girls working in the Waltham Watch Factory were encouraged to learn about the program, which offered them housing and meals in exchange for their apprenticeship training. As experience accumulated in the early years, Charlotte reported that a certificate of physical fitness was added as an admission requirement, along with an age range of twenty-three to thirty-five, good character, and a common school education up to the girl's fifteenth birthday. Since common schools generally teach reading, writing, mathematics, geography, and history, she noted, they were assured that the students could read their textbooks, understand doctors' orders, and read aloud to their patients.

"Our goal in admissions," Charlotte concluded, "is simple: to get the material that will make the finest and most devoted nurses." Charlotte, unsure of Alfred's reaction to her comments, asked if he wished to add anything concerning the Waltham School's admission requirements.

"Thank you, Charlotte. You covered this topic thoroughly," Alfred said.

Recalling their own demanding prerequisite education to college study, Annette, Millie, and Alistair worked to mask their reaction. Rallying first, Annette approached the blackboard. Under Waltham School admission standards, she wrote four broad criteria: age, physical fitness, good character, common school education.

Silence ensued.

Reading the room, Alfred called for a brief break.

As Alfred, Alistair, Charlotte, and Susan sipped iced oolong tea and nibbled on biscuits, Annette and Millie walked to Fay House's backyard, anticipating a long drag on their Vanity Fair cigarettes.

Following her initial reaction, Annette had already begun to sense the liberation emanating from Waltham's admission criteria. If most training schools admit students similarly to Waltham, Annette thought, then we will be at liberty to craft appropriate requirements for admission to a baccalaureate degree program.

Lighting Millie's second cigarette, Annette calmly cautioned her to think of Waltham's lack of defensible admission criteria as a gift to them, one they could advance to achieve their goal.

Following the break, Susan's review of admission criteria to Newark was shorter and more delineated. Established in 1886, one year later than the Waltham School, the Newark School was one of four hospital schools in northern New Jersey. Susan recalled how proud the Newark students were that Clara Weeks, the founding superintendent of the Paterson General Hospital School, had published the first textbook of nursing in 1885 and that the book immediately found a home in their curriculum. Susan was clearly proud of Weeks's book as a product of New Jersey nursing, and everyone knew that it had become widely distributed among newly established training schools.

"In addition to the four requirements of the Waltham School," Susan continued, "my Newark school also mandated that an application form be completed by each candidate." From memory, she recalled some of the nineteen questions. Some were about health: Are you perfectly strong and healthy? Are your sight and hearing perfect? Do you have any physical defects? Have you any uterine complaint? Others were about marital status: Are you single? If a widow, have you children? How are they provided for? Some were about age, height, and weight. Others about past employment. "Lastly," she concluded, "you were asked to promise at all times to obey implicitly the orders of your superior officers." These superior officers, she noted, included doctors and the nursing superintendent.

Annette's suspicions were confirmed.

Remorseless obedience, physical hardiness, and absence of life beyond the hospital and school's walls were key attributes of accepted pupil nurses. She glanced at Alfred, curious about his thoughts. Shifting in his chair, he seemed uncomfortable, as if he wished to be anywhere other than Fay House.

After a brief lunch break of apple, pear, and plum slices with toast and tea, the group refocused, turning to nursing coursework. Annette provided a framework for their discussion, emphasizing the need to define key aspects of a nurse's professional role in health care. "What is the primary role of nurses," she asked the group, "treatment of illness or maintenance of health?" She noted that treatment of disease prioritized the role of doctor's assistant, while management of health signified a broader, more independent role.

"The primary roles of nurses in society will structure the curriculum we outline," Annette said, looking to Alfred for confirmation.

"Indeed, under your framework, the nurse's practice determines coursework," Alfred agreed. Expanding on his statement, he noted that at the Waltham School, as was true for other hospital schools of nursing, graduates take positions in private duty or district nursing. He added that Waltham was significantly different from other schools in one major aspect. Waltham pupils had learning experiences in both home care and hospital care. Other schools focused solely on hospital experiences. Their graduates, however, worked exclusively in homes, environments in which they had no experiences.

Taking charge again, Millie continued the discussion. "If the nurse helps patients maintain health, then what must a pupil nurse learn about health? Health management of an individual, a family, a community, or the general public?"

Shifting roles, Annette now controlled the blackboard, realizing that whomever controlled the chalk had power. On the blackboard, she wrote the heading: *Health means more than lack of disease.*

Charlotte and Susan were first to speak. They emphasized the necessity for a nutrition course to include sick diets and well diets, food guidelines for balanced meals as published in the *Farmers' Bulletin*, meal portion sizes and value of moderate consumption, effects of alcohol, and avoidance of foodborne illnesses. Thoughts spilled out rapidly, without any special order. Annette wrote as quickly as she could, and ideas filled the board: courses on addiction to drugs and alcohol, pain management, physical exercise programs, pregnancy and childbearing, childrearing, childhood markers such as walking and talking, immunizations, dental health, hearing and visual acuity, sexuality and safe sexual practices, signs and symptoms of infection, hazards of immobility, changes with aging, insomnia, and more. Alfred emphasized that the foundation for nursing courses rested on adequate knowledge of biology, chemistry, anatomy, physiology, and mathematics. Millie added culture and religion. Charlotte and Susan nodded their approval.

Lastly, Susan spoke of "common, ever-present mental health disorders, including depression and anxiety, as well as signs of possible suicide." The dam unleashed, Charlotte and Susan spoke for over an hour, outlining essential features of health maintenance without stumbling for words or disagreeing on content. They halted only when Annette's blackboard was completely filled. It was hard to see black behind the chalk. White dust was everywhere, and Annette looked like she had been in a snowstorm.

Then Alfred began to pace in front of the blackboard. He asked if graduates of a Harvard school of nursing could be employed in a hospital. His questions also came rapidly. "Will our new professional nurse learn about surgical techniques? About postoperative management? About complications of surgery and how to avoid such events? About emergency childbirth management? How to deal with treatments for diseases commonly managed in hospitals? Can they be employed by hospitals?"

"If we plan our program well," Annette replied, "then graduates could be employed wherever people exist—homes, hospitals, industry, schools, and other environments. Students could enjoy practice rotations to various general and specialty hospitals, district and visiting nurse associations, industrial clinics, public health departments, and milk stations if so needed."

She proposed that, over the four-year course of their education, students could have experiences in specific medical departments of hospitals and in city dispensaries, missionary shelters, milk stations, and well-baby clinics. Students would learn medical and surgical nursing, obstetrical and gynecological nursing, psychiatric nursing, home care, and community nursing. Nursing students would rotate to sites just as medical students did. The university could expand contracts with hospitals and other agencies to include nursing and medical students.

Alfred stopped pacing. "Yes," he smiled, "that could work!"

Then Alistair began his questions. Focusing on resources, he asked if students would pay tuition and fees comparable to other baccalaureate students, or if they would be financed in other ways, perhaps by hospitals.

The other half of the couple in the bow, Millie answered that tuition and fees would, most likely, be required of all students, unless scholarships become available. Alistair, knowing that they were now rowing together, asked if a nursing school endowment campaign could be undertaken concurrently with the state's approval process. Anticipating the boat's pitch concerning scholarships for women in a nonexistent school, he noted that subtle efforts toward that end could begin sooner rather than later. Funding for a building and personnel salaries might become available as the first class enters. Alistair promised to discuss funding with his father.

As their afternoon progressed rapidly into early evening, the group had etched out a broad definition of baccalaureate nursing and a related scope of practice emanating from a health perspective, along with a four-year course schedule and accompanying diverse practice arrangements. Additionally, they refined admission requirements for consistency with Harvard's standard criteria for baccalaureate education — successful graduation from a public or private four-year high school, including courses in chemistry, biology, mathematics, English, history, and culture. Letters of recommendation and a certificate of health would also be required.

Alfred, realizing that a requirement for chemistry and biology might eliminate candidates whose secondary schools did not offer such courses, suggested that a relationship with Harvard's Lawrence Scientific School be crafted to provide students necessary bridge courses for successful admission to the nursing school. Perhaps a summer program in basic sciences for those seeking admission to nursing, or another program? Quite an attractive and lucrative idea in our gilded age, thought Alfred.

After Alfred spoke, Annette recalled the articles by Charles she had read at the urging of her father. Charles had advocated for change in secondary schools to ensure that graduates could successfully complete radically different curricula in college. Emphasizing educational utility for economic growth and societal advancement, he had called for feeder secondary schools to give students the tools needed for success in specialized college courses.

Rising to the idea of progress, Alfred noted that conversations might begin with the Lawrence Scientific School, as well as neighboring feeder secondary schools. Schools such as the Cambridge School for Girls, still called the Gilmore School, and other private schools might need to revise their curricula to accommodate basic sciences, perhaps even at the expense of classic languages, just as Eliot had predicted.

Annette realized, for the first time as Alfred spoke, that the classics might be collateral damage as their plan evolved.

"We are ready for your and Elizabeth's dinner meeting, Alfred," said Alistair, gleaming confidently at Millie as everyone gathered their belongings to end the day. As the group's scribe, Annette promised to write up the outcomes of their discussions in advance of next week's dinner.

Once goodbyes were said, Annette and Millie returned to their Greek homework, looking forward to reading structured, engaging, and uniformly understood literature.

Greek homework brought pleasant closure to their complex day. But it was Annette alone who wondered if she was responsible for ending the very world she loved.

Meeting conflicts and family emergencies pushed the original ten-day plan for Elizabeth's dinner to mid-October of 1893. The group used this gift of time wisely. They fleshed out their proposal for a four-year baccalaureate nursing program at Harvard, outlining admission criteria, suggested courses, practice rotations, and plans to coordinate with the Lawrence Scientific School and feeder schools.

Extra time also helped Elizabeth Agassiz and Charles in their efforts to galvanize support for degree-granting authority for the Harvard Annex, soon, they hoped, to be called Radcliffe College. Meetings with faculty, alumni, community members, legislators, pastors, and secondary school teachers had been held, resulting in varying degrees of endorsement. As Elizabeth wrote in her diary, "the howl grew louder against Radcliffe" in the late summer and early fall.

Neither Elizabeth Agassiz nor Charles, however, relented in their efforts.

They had fully anticipated opposition.

In late October, Elizabeth and Alfred hosted their dinner party, with Marguerite playing Chopin's Études in the main parlor. Guests were greeted by colorful fall leaves and small pumpkins arranged around the paired arched double doors. Elizabeth and Alfred's home was warm, welcoming, and cheerful. Elizabeth, gracious and elegant in a pale plum-colored evening dress with hair gathered in a lace ribbon to one shoulder, encouraged her guests to take seats at her large dinner table. The subtle aroma of chrysanthemums lingered in both the parlor and dining room.

Entering last, Charles gallantly requested that Elizabeth join him, ushering her forward with a majestic sweep of his hand.

"Behold, Elizabeth Agassiz, soon to be president of Radcliffe College," Charles proclaimed in a resonant voice, theatrically bowing down in front of her. Applause ensued, accompanied by cheers of "Bravo, Lizzie!"

He recounted recent success, emphasizing that Elizabeth had, that very week, won the vote at Harvard to take the proper legal steps to rename the Annex. Forthcoming would be a bill for a college charter to incorporate Radcliffe College. In ceremonious style, Charles led Elizabeth to the head seat at the dining room table. Now overflowing with congratulatory bouquets, Elizabeth delicately moved the flowers to the center of the table and took her seat, glowing with pride.

Charles and Elizabeth had battled over the past few months to secure the vote of the Harvard board and overseers. Despite petitions claiming the demise of quality education if women gained access to higher education, the politically adept pair won their war after they had solidified enough advance assurances to swing the vote.

"The snakes," said Charles coyly as he settled into his own chair, "are nevertheless still in the grass."

The final step, Charles explained to the table as vegetable soup was served, was drafting the Radcliffe College charter, with final approval by the Committee on Education of the Massachusetts Legislature scheduled for February 26th, 1894.

"Negativity remains. Not everyone is a friend," Elizabeth noted. The Association of Collegiate Alumnae had organized in Boston eleven years earlier, she explained, to unite female graduates of four-year colleges and universities on specific issues such as educational standards and economic security of graduates. She noted that the Association's Committee on Endowment of Colleges strongly advocated that any proposed women's college be established only if an adequate endowment had been acquired to ensure that a guarantee of high character be maintained.

"We do not yet have a promised endowment," Elizabeth noted.

"Yet," Charles added. "We are Harvard. Endowments will follow. Any possible concern of the Association of Collegiate Alumnae is no concern of mine." With that, Elizabeth smiled, raised her champagne glass, and thanked everyone present for their commitment to women's education.

Anticipating that the bill of charter for Radcliffe College would pass in winter, Elizabeth looked at Annette and Millie, saying that they would be in the first graduating class in June of 1894.

Imagine that, Annette thought. The first graduating class at Radcliffe College.

Decision

Handling John Billings's letter reverently, Alfred carefully slid his sterling silver letter opener, a gift from his mother when he began his medical practice, in the envelope, removing the single sheet gently. Dated November 1893, Billings's short letter informed Alfred of a meeting of superintendents of training schools for nurses scheduled for January 10, 1894, at the Academy of Medicine in New York City.

Billings, Alfred's icon, was brief in his letter:

> *Nursing superintendents of training schools attached to general hospitals in the United States and Canada are organizing to standardize educational programs. While your hospital is relatively new and growing, it is a general hospital with a nursing school. You must send your superintendent to this meeting. I have been asked by Miss Anna L. Alston, superintendent of Mount Sinai Training School for Nursing in New York City and current president of the temporary organization established in June during the Congress of Nurses at the World's Fair, to forward names and addresses of superintendents to invite to the January meeting.*

The letter ended with a complimentary close, and simple advice.

Be in the tent on this one, Alfred.

Included also was a single postscript.

The announcement of this meeting was published in the October 1893 issue of The Trained Nurse and Hospital Review.

Alfred placed Billings's letter on his desk. Yes, he decided, Charlotte Macleod must attend the January meeting. I will let Charlotte know to expect an invitation from Miss Alston, he thought, putting a reminder on his calendar.

Alfred had not seen the announcement. Neither the hospital nor the school received *The Review*, a new journal established in 1889 and published by Lakeside Publishing in New York. Covering a broad range of subjects as diverse as injection techniques and hospital security, the journal was a popular vehicle for communications among nurses and hospital administrators. We must subscribe to this journal, Alfred thought, making a mental note.

Swept up in Charles's planning activities surrounding women and Harvard, Alfred found the letter from Billings provocative. While he no longer felt sandwiched between the ethos of the Nightingale-era nursing-controlled schools and the efficiency of hospitalism using pupil nurses as cheap labor, he found that the letter would put his new convictions to the test.

Is the Waltham Hospital considered a general hospital—at least in the sense implied by nurse leaders? A general hospital, he recalled, was one not specializing in treatment of a specific disease or illness. Knowing that writing always sharpened his mind, Alfred placed paper and his new fountain pen on his desk, prepared to outline Waltham Hospital's chronology, a comforting activity.

The Waltham Training School for Nurses was established in 1885, three years before the hospital was officially opened for patient care. In the first years of the school, pupil nurses apprenticed doctors on home visits and assisted the nursing superintendent and her assistant in district nursing. Local physicians and the nursing superintendent provided weekly lectures. Pupil nurses soon realized that severely ill patients warranted hospital care, not home care. In that early period, however, such sick patients traveled by train or horse-drawn carriage to either neighboring cities for hospital care or to the poor farm, depending on their resources.

The nursing school demanded the establishment of a hospital in Waltham.

What an anomaly, thought Alfred, smiling to himself. A school needing a hospital.

Due to failed efforts to secure an endowment, Waltham Hospital delayed opening until 1888. In the interim, Alfred's friend Edward R. Cutler, in a haze of cigar smoke, transformed his large home into Waltham's first general hospital in 1885, accommodating four patients as well as the nursing school. Called the Cutler Hospital, this early facility proved invaluable to the community. Renovated in 1887, it was outfitted for fifteen adult beds and two cribs. Edward leased the expanded facility, now called the Waltham Cottage Hospital, to a new hospital board and the Waltham Training School for Nurses, with nursing services to be provided by the school. Only one year later, the Waltham Cottage Hospital was incorporated as the Waltham Hospital, with a new cost-sharing agreement drawn between the hospital and the school.

We moved quickly, thought Alfred.

While chronic cases were not admitted to Waltham Hospital, cases of incipient tuberculosis were admitted, pending space availability, to receive currently used treatment protocols. An accident room, with closets for instruments, medicines, and surgical supplies, was constructed with easy ramp access direct to the main front doors. A small surgical outpatient area was added adjacent to the accident room. Additionally, the pest house, previously used for the care of contagious patients, was thoroughly cleaned and established as the hospital's contagious department one year later.

In 1892, the Waltham Hospital board, overwhelmed with demands from doctors and community residents for additional patient beds, relocated to a new, larger building one mile from the Waltham Training School for Nurses, which remained in the previously expanded Waltham Hospital. The school and hospital boasted both a superintendent and a matron, respectively, along with separate buildings, marking their relative independence. Now, one year later, thought Alfred proudly, the hospital has rented an adjacent tenement, allowing for care of five or six nervous cases on a regular basis. Deeply committed to Waltham, the hospital and school also provided direct services to baby milk stations and factories, including the Waltham Watch Factory.

Satisfied that he had chronicled the history well, Alfred identified Waltham as a general hospital, and thus, eligible to participate in the newly forming association of superintendents of training schools.

Offering general hospital services as well as specific specialties, home care, district nursing, and other community services, surely, thought Alfred, the Waltham School would exceed the expectations of any new nursing association.

Perhaps, in New York, Charlotte might visit Lucy L. Drown, superintendent at the Boston City Hospital Training School for Nurses, for an update on efforts to organize superintendents of training schools. Drown would surely be in New York. Since she had not attended the June Congress of Nurses in Chicago, Charlotte might benefit from an update from a superintendent of a school operational for almost twenty years. Alfred hoped to mitigate Charlotte's naivety concerning the politics of nursing administrators.

His mind wandering, Alfred recalled his experiences with Linda Richards, appointed superintendent of the Boston Training School for Nurses during his last year at Harvard Medical School. Alfred, in charge of both obstetrics and nursing services at Boston's Lying-In Hospital at that time, would occasionally come in contact with Richards, with whom he developed a professional relationship. Drawing on his relationship with her, Alfred decided to introduce himself and Charlotte Macleod to Lucy Drown in his letter, asking that she update Charlotte on current events regarding nursing organizations.

Pleased with his efforts, Alfred believed it would be excellent for Charlotte to have a colleague at the January nursing meeting in New York.

Yet, he also knew that interpretation of the phrase "standardize educational programs" would determine who would, and who would not, remain colleagues.

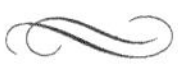

Amidst a brief flurry of snow, Charlotte braced herself against twenty-five-degree temperature and howling winds as she stepped from the two-seat hansom cab onto Third Street in Lower Manhattan. The cab took her from the Cortlandt Street Ferry Depot to the nearby rail line, a short but heavily congested distance. The Third Avenue Elevated Line, or the Third Avenue EL, constructed in 1878, ran from South Ferry at Battery Park in Lower Manhattan to Harlem in Upper Manhattan. Wrapping her woolen scarf around her neck and pulling her woolen beret forward and down over her ears, Charlotte hopped on the train, tucking her large carpetbag on the floor between her knees for safety.

The short six-mile trip to Grand Central Depot at Forty-Second Street and Park Avenue was delicious to Charlotte. She found the depot impressive, constructed in red pressed brick with cast-iron trim, designed by architect John Snook as an example of the American Second Empire style, with a roof of iron and glass. Recognized as a mammoth, majestic building symbolic of America's economic growth, the depot screamed industry and wealth.

I am far from Waltham and my room at the training school, Charlotte thought.

She had traveled most of the day, and now the sun was beginning to set over the Manhattan skyline. She stopped for a moment to watch a blaze of yellow descend below the gray buildings, the branchless trees standing silently with her as night fell. She was delighted to be here, in this moment, at this place.

A newcomer to Manhattan, Charlotte disembarked from the Third Avenue EL train at Grand Central Depot and walked the remainder of her journey to her destination, the Hotel Brunswick, about fifteen blocks away on Fifth Avenue between Twenty-Sixth and Twenty-Seventh Streets. At the juncture between Madison Square Park and Fifth Avenue, the hotel, designed for conferences and visitors, was a welcome site. Elegant and ornate, the hotel advertised fashionable guest rooms with adjoining bathrooms, several restaurants, and shops on the street level. A stay at the Brunswick would be an expensive treat, and she was thankful to Alfred for funding her expenses.

Irrespective of the opulence, however, Charlotte had doubts.

Despite Alfred's charming introductory letter to Lucy Drown, Charlotte was denied a personal meeting with the Boston City Hospital superintendent of nurses in a chilly letter:

Dear Ms. Macleod,

Due to my current responsibilities at the Boston City Hospital Training School for Nurses, as well as my preparation for the upcoming First Annual Convention, I cannot meet with you at this time.

I look forward to meeting you at the convention, if you plan to attend.

Sincerely,

Miss Lucy Drown

Although Drown's message was curt, Charlotte was not offended and still wanted to explore the nursing program at Boston City Hospital.

In reviewing the 1891 published report of the Boston City Hospital Training School for Nurses prior to arriving in New York, Charlotte had begrudgingly found herself impressed. Since its inception in 1878, the school had graduated 242 nurses, with thirty completing the program in 1890. Contrary to the Waltham School's pattern of practice rotations involving hospital care as well as home and district care, the Boston program pamphlet claimed that "two full years, under the best of conditions, with a fixed and continuous course of study and drill, and *the whole amount of time given to hospital work*, is none too much for one who claims to be a well-trained nurse."

Assuming Miss Drown as the author of the pamphlet, Charlotte noted that the Boston superintendent frowned on sending pupil nurses to private-duty nursing cases, stating that financial gain to small hospitals from such practice is "at the expense of the best care of hospital patients." Charlotte saw this statement as a double standard, given that pupil nurses routinely cared for hospital patients in order for hospitals to avoid the expense of employing graduate nurses. This ubiquitous practice, common to hospitals with training schools, however, did not draw criticism—at least, she thought, not yet.

In reading the application form, also included in the pamphlet, Charlotte noted that applicants were mandated to attest to their strength, general health, lack of physical defects, perfect sight and hearing, freedom from domestic responsibilities, and completion of basic education. The militaristic orientation of the program was sobering, with day duty described as eleven hours, with one hour for rest after 2:00 pm, one half day off each week, and four hours free on Sundays. The tone of the pamphlet, as well as the content, was mechanistic to Charlotte.

Charlotte interpreted the tone toward pupil nurses at the Boston School as cold and uncaring, but struggled to remain gracious in her thoughts toward Lucy Drown, allowing for mistakes sometimes made in the uncertainty attendant to relatively new ventures. In time and with exposure to practices of other superintendents, thought Charlotte, Lucy would be exposed to new ideas, thus possibly changing her drill and kill practice.

Charlotte awoke on Wednesday, January 10th, 1894, anticipating a new and exciting venture in a community of nursing colleagues. Others in health, she knew, enjoyed similar community. In 1847, the American Medical Association was established by physicians to "promote the art and science of medicine," launching the *Journal of the American Medical Association* in 1883 for dissemination of medical news and scientific advancements. Likewise, the American Public Health Association, founded in 1872, was organized to support the work of public health professionals in managing communicable and other diseases. And now, she thought, walking briskly from the Hotel Brunswick to the Academy of Medicine at 17 West Forty-Third Street, we will have a place of our own in this timely venture for a nursing organization.

Undaunted by the frigid weather, Charlotte felt warm. Her spirits high, she admired the Academy's building, constructed in 1890 with five floors of conference rooms and a large medical library. While she enjoyed the cobblestone streets outside the building and the occasional flagstone crosswalk, Charlotte heard several conversations that they would soon be converted to asphalt, a much less charming appearance. She was also taken by the signage inside the building regarding the Academy's suggestion to the New York City Common Council to establish the Metropolitan Board of Health, the first such public health establishment in the country. Impressed by the Academy's initiatives, Charlotte looked forward to her organization's future ventures.

Cloaked in the charms of New York City and the Academy, Charlotte entered the prestigious building with both respect and excitement. After checking in at the registration table and receiving her name tag, she selected a seat in the conference room.

The meeting started promptly at 10:00 am. Anna L. Alston, president of the temporary organization previously established during the June Congress of Nurses, presided. Alston indicated that seventy-one invitations to attend the convention were mailed to superintendents of representative schools attached to general hospitals. Of these, she reported, thirty responded positively to the invitation. Charlotte was one of the thirty invitees present. A small, highly charged group, thought Charlotte.

With pen in hand, Charlotte jotted notes concerning the first action item—the organization's constitution and bylaws. The materials had been previously developed by a committee to draft resolutions, constituted during the June Congress of Nurses. As each article of these documents was read, discussion ensued with amendments made to final versions. Charlotte was particularly fascinated with the phrase "training schools connected with incorporated and well-organized general hospitals," with programs giving at least two years' course of instruction. After the amended constitution and bylaws were endorsed, the question of the size and importance which a training school should attain before finding representation through its superintendent in the Society of Superintendents was actively discussed. Five members, including Drown, were selected by Alston to serve on an eligibility committee to address this matter, with a report to be given at the Second Annual Convention in 1895.

Although a committee had been constituted to address eligibility, lively, at times passionate, discussion accompanied the topic of hospital size. Participants discussed the need for specific rotations in medical departments, assuming that the sponsoring hospital had a sufficient number of beds to provide thorough and practical experiences in these branches. Given that participants agreed that teaching needed to be given only in hospitals over a two-year course of practice, they discussed the possibility of lengthening programs to three years in hospitals with insufficient cases to address this deficiency. Some advanced the idea that hospitals with less than 150 beds might require three years of training rather than two years. Tangential topics such as preliminary qualifications, textbooks, examinations, and other details of training were also briefly discussed.

The meeting adjourned at 5:00 pm, with participants invited to a parting dinner at the Hotel Brunswick to honor the occasion of the Society's establishment. Following dinner, Charlotte sought Lucy Drown, wishing to finally introduce herself to another Massachusetts superintendent. While Lucy shook Charlotte's hand, her facial expression was flat, bordering on condescending.

"Do you believe you will join this organization?" Lucy asked.

"Yes, I am eager to!" Charlotte waited for a reply.

"Will your hospital meet requirements for support of an adequate training school?" Lucy questioned in a tone that seemed to border on condescension and interrogation.

"Why, yes, we will certainly meet, and perhaps exceed, requirements for an excellent school," Charlotte said proudly. "Even Miss Florence Nightingale has complimented our training program."

"Miss Nightingale does not lead American nursing, Miss Macleod," exclaimed Lucy flatly, dropping Charlotte's hand. With an almost imperceptible shake of her head, Lucy turned from Charlotte without saying goodbye.

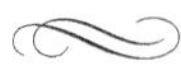

"Tell me, how did you enjoy Gotham?" Annette, preparing the kitchen table at Fay House for a light breakfast meeting with Alfred and Charlotte, lightly bantered with Charlotte about her impressions of New York City.

"Gotham?" Charlotte asked.

"Gotham is a nickname for New York City," Annette explained. Expanding on the name, she said that Washington Irving, a writer, mockingly called New York City Gotham in an 1807 issue of the satirical magazine *Salmagundi*. Irving likened New York City to the people of Gotham in England, who, Annette said, he had claimed were absurdly mad.

"My father is a newspaper journalist. He now works for *The Boston Globe*, but when we lived in New York, he was an editorial writer for *The New York Times*. I learned a great deal from him about Manhattan."

As Annette placed warm scones and raspberry jam on delicate China dessert plates, Alfred rushed into the room, stating that he was late because a sick patient had needed his care.

"Alfred," said Annette slowly, "you can only blame your patients so many times before we will stop believing you." Laughing with Charlotte, Annette pulled out a chair for him at the table.

"Touch the scones," Annette said, "they are still warm. You are not that late."

As they drafted a bare-bones curriculum for a four-year nursing degree program at Harvard, Alfred and Annette knew that a key task was to understand programs currently offered at hospital training schools for nurses. They both turned to Charlotte to launch their discussion.

"Tell us what you learned at the conference, Charlotte," said Annette.

Since the conference was held two weeks ago, Charlotte had time to objectively digest training school programs described as ideal by the superintendents present. Her summary was simple: First, best programs were those offered by general hospitals with multiple services and adequate bed capacity for pupil nurses' training. Second, a minimum of two consecutive years of hospital training with a uniform, fixed curriculum regulated by state boards of examiners, was considered mandatory.

Charlotte noted that, in multiple discussions, it was stated that training was to be in hospitals and not in patients' homes. She added that private-duty experiences were considered unnecessary if adequate training in hospitals was offered, assuming that graduate nurses could easily generalize learning to different situations. Furthermore, it was considered unethical to accept income from care given by pupil nurses in homes, even if given under supervision of a superintendent.

"No one, however, argued that hospitals should enjoy daily, around-the-clock free services from pupil nurses treated, at best, as voiceless indentured domestic servants bound by application agreements." Charlotte added that the superintendents believed their first obligation is to the hospital, and secondly, to pupil nurses.

She added with emphasis, "The *patient first principle* is an assumed obligation."

"As well," she continued, "Lucy Drown will not be at one with us."

"I have had time to consider our own Waltham program over the past few weeks, and I must say that I would appreciate your consideration of changes in it, Alfred." Faced with a new perspective, particularly one framed in a backdrop of efforts for women's education and suffrage, Charlotte felt distraught and used. Why should nurses settle for arduous apprenticeship training rather than college education?

"Like you, Charlotte," Alfred said, "I have also recently changed my thoughts about nurses' education. We will certainly make changes. I am committed to that end with you."

"For now, however, we must focus on our presentation for the planning team, after the upcoming hearing before the Committee on Education of the Massachusetts Legislature at the statehouse set for February the 28th," Annette added firmly. "Change will happen," she assured both Charlotte and Alfred. "But," she said, "first things first — let's craft a curriculum suitable for a college degree."

With blackboard at her back and chalk in hand, Annette returned to her task of scribing their work. She had always loved the smell of chalk.

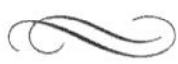

"In a general sense, a four-year curriculum for a nursing degree might be modeled after a four-year medical degree program," Alfred offered, waving a copy of the *Annual Catalogue of the Medical School 1893-1894* in his left hand. The ninety-four-page catalogue provided relevant information concerning the medical curriculum that most interested them, including requirements for admission, methods of instruction, textbooks, clinical practice sites, examinations, library resources, pecuniary aid, tuition, and fees. For Annette, perhaps the most revealing section of the catalogue was the distribution of courses per week, per day, per hour, per four years of classes. Like farmers, she thought, medical students worked from see to can't see.

For Annette, the catalogue was thrilling, a regimen projecting assurance and confidence.

For Charlotte, the catalogue was an epiphany. In medical schools, student education was the first principle.

If nurse leaders were linking state nursing registration to hospital size, bed capacity, and service departments, then thoroughly recognizing the varied rotations of medical students to clinical agencies in the Boston area was critical. Alfred summarized what were termed in the catalogue as the "clinical advantages of the school," given its location in a large, progressive city with multiple general as well as specialty facilities. Among them, Alfred read in rapid succession the Massachusetts General Hospital, Boston City Hospital, Boston Lying-In Hospital, Boston Dispensary, Massachusetts Charitable Eye and Ear Infirmary, Marine Hospital at Chelsea, Free Hospital for Women, Children's Hospital, and Carney Hospital. Students rotated to various clinical services, both in the hospital and in outpatient departments.

"Since the medical school already has agreements with these facilities for medical student rotations, I imagine that legal agreements for nursing student rotations can be crafted to mirror similar arrangements for pupil nurses." Smiling, Alfred noted that such affiliations would negate concerns about possible deficiencies in clinical experiences due to inadequate cases in small hospitals.

One particular fourth-year rotation amazed Annette and Charlotte. They found the mandatory rotation to the Boston Cooking School twice weekly for one month curious. Do these students cook? Annette wondered. Are they expected to cook? questioned Charlotte. The Boston Cooking School, established in 1879 by the Women's Education Association of Boston, provided instruction in cooking to those who wanted to earn their living as cooks.

"Good nutrition is important to both health and recovery from illness," Charlotte added. "But learning to cook is questionable. Perhaps we can consider a course in nutrition rather than an entire rotation in the hospital kitchen." Charlotte recalled that when she had provided home care, she had frequent conversations with mothers about balancing diets, providing tips on how to plan diets, even when money was scarce. Rolling her eyes and sighing, Charlotte also lamented the "frighteningly poor dental health of so many of my patients," often related to excessive sweets and lack of regular toothbrushing. Now on a tangent, Charlotte suggested that perhaps nutrition and dental care could be combined in a single course, given the relationship between them.

"We can have a major impact with a course such as this. Given that tube toothpaste and improved toothbrushes only became available in 1892, this type of course would combine science with practical technology." Charlotte spoke hurriedly, excited about the real possibility of creating a curriculum centered on daily health.

"Perhaps," Annette said, "the underlying importance of balanced nutrition and food types might be taught, with teaching of cooking left to cooks to teach their students. Maybe a short experience in a hospital kitchen to observe food essentials, such as food storage, meal preparation, estimation of freshness, and portion sizes." Thinking of her experience in home care in Waltham, Annette offered that such observational experience might be particularly valuable for private-duty nurses or those working in public health.

"Domestic science," Alfred offered, "might include cooking and the other ideas you both mentioned." He noted that home management, or home economics, was "quite the rage in America," with programs teaching cooking, sewing, home finance, childcare, cleaning and laundry, and other topics. Courses in domestic arts and sciences were now offered in high schools and even some colleges.

"Since our probationary period focuses on home management, I wonder if we should include such a course in the nursing program we are designing." Charlotte asked Annette to place home economics, or domestic science, on the blackboard.

"We will have no difficulty designing our college curriculum *if* we first get a good handle on the practice of nursing," Alfred reminded his colleagues.

"What do nurses do?"

Silence followed his simple question. Annette recalled the instrumentalism of Aristotle, his means-to-an-end logic. She knew the next line of thought would get them efficiently to the curriculum content.

What do I do as a doctor? Alfred thought as they stopped for lunch.

They munched on peanut butter and jelly sandwiches, two treats first introduced, Alfred recalled, by Ambrose Straub and Charles Welch during the 1893 World's Fair. While the peanut butter left Annette with a gooey taste in her mouth, she enjoyed every morsel of her sandwich.

As they ate, Alfred asked if it might help if he described what he did as a doctor. His stream-of-consciousness flow impressed Annette, who had become acquainted with the phrase made popular by psychologist William James.

"First, I collect information. Does my patient have a complaint? What is that complaint? Then, I examine the patient, especially the area where the problem presents. Irrespective of complaints, I generally listen to my patient's heart and lungs, sounds from these organs being vital. Once I come to my diagnosis, I decide on treatment. Sometimes I send my patient to a specialist for additional evaluation and treatment." He further explained that he intermittently saw patients after the original treatment to evaluate follow-up progress and to decide if new treatments were needed. His musings got the conversation going.

"Charlotte, and also Alfred, let's now turn to what nurses do, and I'll jot these functions on the blackboard. Let's begin with Alfred's mention of treatment." Annette stood by the portable blackboard, chalk in hand.

Seeking clarification, Charlotte asked if she should address functions that only nurses could do, eliminating those tasks routinely completed by nurses but more appropriately ascribed to others, including cooks, housemaids, laundresses, and domestic servants. Seeing both Alfred and Annette nod their heads affirmatively, Charlotte rose and began listing nursing functions.

"While we carry out doctors' treatments both in hospitals and homes, we also administer medications, manage surgical dressing sites, provide anesthesia in surgical suites, assist in progressive ambulation and range-of-joint motion exercises, deliver babies if needed, administer immunizations, teach women pregnancy care and infant care, and perform other functions for maintaining the public's health." With a sweep of her hand in the air above her, Charlotte smiled, stating that the outline would scrape the surface of nurses' work.

"I believe that our most important work is education," Charlotte added as she returned to her seat and sipped her tea. Summarizing, Charlotte mentioned that nurses teach new mothers about baby and childcare; offer comfort to depressed and anxious patients; explain infectious diseases, including signs and symptoms as well as treatments; describe effects of alcoholism and drug addiction on both the patient and family; encourage participation in immunization programs; instruct primarily women on nutritious diets and quality food choices; and much more.

"What nurses do can easily fill a four-year college nursing program," Charlotte confidently declared.

"Alfred, do you wish to add anything?" asked Annette.

"I can only add that eliminating work better done by others will elevate nursing, allowing it visibility as a profession."

Alfred sat quietly, shaking his head.

"How were Edward Cutler, the other Waltham Hospital board members, and I so blind when we originally structured our training program? We expected our pupil nurses to assume multiple jobs, and to do those jobs quietly, submissively, without the enjoyment of a typical American home life."

"Hospitalism is a national movement.," Annette replied. "You were swept up in it. The hospital is the nurses' convent, the doctor her deity. The enterprise generated money and improved doctors' lifestyles."

Annette was desperate to end their work on a more pleasant, high note. A wounded Alfred was of no use to them.

"We are today's change agents. We can free nurses from monasticism and assert their role in patient care, not simply obedience to doctors. Our work will allow doctors to focus attention on disease management, and nurses on health and restoration, with education an essential tool." Raising her teacup, Annette predicted that the outcomes of their work would be admired by their colleagues.

Taking Alfred aside at the end of their meeting, Annette thanked him for his honesty and courage.

"I very much respect your comments this afternoon. Something great will come from our work, Alfred. Your resolute commitment to nursing practice has the potential to refocus all of us on health, not simply elimination of disease. Thank you."

Smiling, Alfred put on his overcoat and left from the front door. Annette knew that Alfred, a powerful figure fraught with worry and ambiguity, would need little help to retain his heartfelt commitment. Yet his vision, she also knew, remained clouded by guilt.

"Surely you are not serious, Alfred," Henry Wood had commented, cheeks flushing red as he glared at his friend.

The meeting Alfred and Millie were having with board members of the Waltham Hospital and Waltham Training School for Nurses was not going well. Apart from Edward Cutler, the initial response of the five other board members was horror. Dr. Wood was beyond himself.

The meeting had begun well enough. Since the same people composed both the Waltham Hospital and the Waltham Hospital Training School boards, including all original founding doctors, Alfred had focused his introductory remarks broadly on education of women in America during their initial meeting. He reviewed the history of the Harvard Annex, informing them of current efforts by Charles Eliot and Elizabeth Agassiz to secure degree-granting authority for the women's college.

Juxtaposing the training school's program and structure against college programs, specifically comparing Harvard Medical School to the Waltham nursing school, Alfred emphasized that apprenticeship training in a hospital did not equate with education in a college setting.

"Hospitals provide care for patients. Colleges provide education for students. If what nurses do is important to patient care, why would nursing students be educated in a manner different from doctors? One reason. Hospital thralldom demands obedient servitude from pupil nurses, akin to slavery, to ensure hospital income. Our oppressive system is wrong. We must change our program. Nurses must be educated, just like dentists, engineers, doctors, and others."

And that, precisely, is where the boat began to list to the starboard side.

"Henry, we are in Massachusetts, the country's leader in college education," replied Alfred, hoping to right the boat. "Yet we operate nurses' training programs," he continued, "as if pupils are church deaconesses living in the eighteenth century, constrained to serve for consecutive years in hospitals, their education, such as we give them, only when patient needs are first met."

"I am embarrassed, Henry, that I have only recently come to this understanding, primarily through the efforts of Charles and Elizabeth regarding women's education." Silent after this statement, Alfred had turned to Edward Cutler, inviting him to speak.

"I agree with Alfred, and I know that this topic is frightening. Who will care for patients in hospitals if pupils are not always on duty? Can we afford to pay graduate nurses? Will we be called more frequently to see hospitalized patients? On a personal note, will we lose income? Will our lives change?"

Alfred, impatient with the limited views of his colleagues, including Edward, whose questions seemed to fuel the fire, turned the conversation to change, encouraging board members to advocate for change, recalling the glory and glamor of the World's Fair, held only months earlier, a fair advancing America as the world's global leader.

Tasked by Alfred to compose specific questions, board members calmed. As the meeting proceeded, Alfred realized how clever his old friend had been. Once those questions of self-interest were raised, they could be directly answered. Alfred saw the gleam in Edward's eye as he sipped his coffee, lit his cigar, and watched the adventure begin.

After several hours of lively conversation, a straw vote to approve the transition of the training school to a college program was unanimously endorsed. Members then moved from the conference room to an adjacent parlor room at Waltham Hospital, sipping tea and coffee as they discussed the recent development of sickness funds offered both by banks and various industries, intended to offset charges of doctors and hospitals when patients were unable to work. Several members knew of efforts to organize hospital administrators, an endeavor to establish a trade group unifying various diverse hospitals and care networks for business purposes. Perhaps also useful for cost savings and rate setting.

Focusing on what would impact physicians, Edward had truly saved the day. Looking at his old friend surrounded by good colleagues and enlivening conversation, Alfred imagined that Edward was glad to have left his sheltered front porch.

At fifty-seven years of age, Arthur Gilman was a spry, energetic man, sporting a walrus-style mustache with side-parted hair that characteristically curled over his ears. On the chilly but sunny morning of Wednesday, February 28, 1894, Arthur, wearing a dark steel-gray cotton inverness cloak and black leather lace boots, gleamed with confidence and pride. Escorting Elizabeth Agassiz, his left arm locked over her right arm, Arthur, generally loquacious, seemed lost for words.

While never chatty herself, Elizabeth did not share Arthur's confidence today.

"Arthur," she whispered, "remember that we cannot predict the outcome today."

For almost two decades, Arthur and Elizabeth had worked tirelessly to secure college education for women. Today, the Committee on Education of the Massachusetts Legislature would meet at the statehouse to hear arguments either to support, or deny, a bill to charter the Harvard Annex as Radcliffe College, with degree-granting authority.

Elizabeth, a realist, had prepared herself for all possible outcomes. Understanding the importance of appearance, she wore a crimson-colored shawl over a lace-frilled white blouse and a full-length black satin Eudora skirt. She was regal, dressed in a hint of Harvard color. As she and Arthur approached the statehouse, Elizabeth, taken with the gilded dome of the original red-brick Bulfinch building, was momentarily overwhelmed by the magnitude of their bill. Educating women, she thought, is comparable to freeing slaves. Erosion of oppression. While Charles had briefed his crew members to avoid any mention of suffrage, Elizabeth, like Charles and Arthur, knew that education would fling open many doors, forever changing the American landscape.

Today, however, Elizabeth was grounded, knowing the opposition slithered, ready to strike down their bill. She again cautioned Arthur to brace for possible disappointment, a caution she did not need to share with Charles, who had weathered many similar legislative battles over the past twenty-five years.

Knowing that news reporters would cover the event, disseminating the outcome to the general public, Charles invited several influential people to the legislative meeting. Among them, Amos and Caroline Fiske, who accepted his invitation graciously, as did Claire Williams, president of the Boston region for the General Federation of Women's Club. Alistair and his father, Matthew, as well as several representatives of Harvard's alumni and select graduate and undergraduate Annex students also agreed to attend.

Charles knew that legislators revered Harvard professors. Despite his occasional misgivings regarding the validity of this reverence, Charles had periodically capitalized on it for the benefit of Harvard. Conferring with Elizabeth and Arthur, Charles invited several of the original thirty-eight Harvard faculty who had volunteered to teach Annex students in 1879 to participate in the hearing, including James B. Greenough, Le Baron Russell Briggs, William W. Goodwin, and George Herbert Palmer. Charles and Elizabeth, knowing that these highly respected educators could substantiate the academic success of students who had been awarded certificates, would negate a popular notion, often repeated, that "Annex girls are flighty students."

Annette, Millie, Alfred, and Alistair, accompanied by Charlotte, served as essential staff for Charles and Elizabeth, each ready to provide prepared testimony, if called upon. Otherwise, they rotated through the conference room, updating Charles and Elizabeth on attendees, transmitting overheard gossip, highlighting opponents, and performing other generally useful staff tasks. Charles had warned his crew to refrain from conversations regarding suffrage, alcoholic temperance, or anti-lynching, since such would blend issues, derail the bill, and increase opposition.

"Whatever you do, don't waste time with advocates," Charles cautioned. "They are already on our side."

Like Elizabeth, Charles's crew members had dressed for the occasion, each wearing crimson accessories, Alfred and Alistair with Harvard ties, Annette with crimson silk ribbon wove through her long braid, and Millie and Charlotte each wearing crimson brooches borrowed from Elizabeth. The conference room originally selected for the hearing was replaced with a larger one, at the request of Arthur, who informed the government staff member that the number of speakers for the hearing, as well as the number of audience participants, mandated more space and additional seating. While Annette had wished for the meeting to be held in the rotunda, she was nonetheless impressed by the stateliness of the building, as well as the current expansion designed by Charles Brigham. The building felt royal, final. Recalling Oliver Wendell Holmes's nickname for the statehouse as the "Hub of the Solar System" and Boston as the "Hub of the Universe," Annette smiled to herself, thinking that perhaps, just this once, women would win the day.

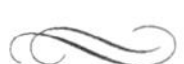

Opponents to the bill were varied, with many signed up to provide verbal testimony. Major opposition came from the Association of Collegiate Alumnae, an organization founded in 1882 to unite women graduates of four-year colleges and universities on issues surrounding standards for academic programs. The Committee on Endowment of this organization highly objected to the passage of the Radcliffe bill, stating that the institution was without adequate endowment to ensure a guarantee of high character maintained. Members of the Collegiate Alumnae, as well as current students of six women's degree-granting colleges and universities, inundated the Massachusetts legislature and Harvard's president and fellows with opposition protest letters.

The day prior to the hearing, Arthur Gilman had invited Ellen Richards, a founding member of the Association of Collegiate Alumnae, to consult with her about the situation. Her opposition, she informed him politely, was the very best thing that could be done for her sex. While they disagreed, Arthur invited his guest to withdraw her opposition nevertheless, which she refused to do. At the hearing, Ellen Richards sat at a table supported on either side by attorneys.

Calling the hearing to order, the chairman of the Committee on Education asked each side to present their views. Without any pre-planning, attendees at the hearing sat together in two groups, the *groom's side*, on the left, represented the Radcliffe College advocates, while the *bride's side*, on the right, represented opponents to the bill. A member of the Harvard Corporation made a plain statement: "We intend to give to women the same instruction that men have so long enjoyed. The charter is being asked in order that the Annex might be permanently established, and be authoritatively carried on with the aid of the president and fellows of Harvard College."

Elizabeth then gave details of the Annex's past work, as well as plans for the growth of the college. William W. Goodwin, professor of Greek, then compared the female mind of his Annex students favorably to his male students, emphasizing the economical merits of the bill. When Charles stood at the podium, the room quieted. Very aware of his own influence, Charles, indicating that Harvard was the active agent at the hearing, reviewed how the institution had "widened its scope of activity by taking up instruction in law, in medicine, in whatever else" it deemed appropriate for the country. He concluded his brief remarks by leaning forward at the podium, looking intensely at the committee members, asking one emphatic question:

"If Harvard College takes up the education of women, is there any reason to suppose that it will ever renounce it?"

Silence.

When asked to provide testimony, opponents to the bill spoke of lack of endowment, lack of trust in Harvard's commitment to Radcliffe College, and general disagreement that Harvard needed to engage in women's education. Following all presentations, committee members heard from the senior attorney representing Ellen Richards.

Rising from his chair, he said that his client had withdrawn all opposition to the bill. After a brief recess, committee members returned and announced approval of the Radcliffe College bill. Although the official meeting was then closed, the committee chairman expressed his admiration for Elizabeth.

"I'd like to do anything that lady wants me to do. She must be the head of this proposed Radcliffe College."

The senior attorney for the opposition, speaking privately to Arthur after the hearing, indicated that he would donate his legal fees provided by his client to Radcliffe College, given his impressions of Elizabeth Agassiz.

Goal one, the award of degree-granting authority to Radcliffe College, had been accomplished. Governor Frederic Greenhalge signed the act of incorporation for the college on March 23, 1894. This act stated that

> *Radcliffe College is hereby authorized to confer on women all honors and degrees as fully as any university or college in this commonwealth is now so empowered respecting men or women:*

provided, however, that no degree shall be conferred by the said Radcliffe College except with the approval of the president and fellows of Harvard College, given on satisfactory evidence of such qualification as is accepted for the same degree when conferred by Harvard University.

As the hearing adjourned, dusk fell, with people slowly leaving the State House. Charles's crew assembled under the seven arches of the front terrace, waiting for him before advancing to the four tiers of steps to Beacon Street.

"Congratulations everyone!" Charles beamed, taking Elizabeth's hand in his.

"Women may now be college educated, awarded Radcliffe College degrees. We may now press our second goal, the establishment of a Harvard school of nursing, possibly a more taxing part of our journey together."

Walking down the tiered steps, his crew following, he turned to them as he approached his hansom cab, congratulating them again.

"We will meet on Monday, March 26th, in my office at seven am. Be prompt."

Given the time of day, Annette watched the statehouse's gilded dome glisten against the setting sun.

Now part of history, women had a place in Cambridge.

The first line on Charles's March 26th, 1894, agenda read:

"7:00 am to 7:10 am, Joy and Jubilation."

Crimson-colored roses adorned the center of Charles's large conference table. His crew, seated at the table, were eager to revel in their statehouse victory.

For ten minutes.

"Congratulations for your efforts. It was the right cause, the right time. We succeeded. Now, we move to a more difficult task. Health care is treacherous. Sly, rapacious opponents lurk behind closed doors. Greed trumps goodwill."

As Charles closed the door to the conference room, Annette briefly saw her mother and father walking briskly down the hall to the room.

Amos knocked.

"Our meeting began at 7:00 am. Do you wish to join us?" asked Charles, eyebrows raised. Apologizing for being a few minutes late, Amos retrieved several documents from his weathered sixteen-inch ox-leather Gladstone bag.

Below the fold in *The Globe* on Sunday, March 25th, 1894, a headline read: *Governor Greenhalge Signs Act of Incorporation for Radcliffe College.* Amos distributed copies of the newspaper to everyone at the table, beginning with Charles. In the article, Amos had briefly summarized the evolution of the Harvard Annex to the college, with appealing descriptions of key players in the drama. Characterizing Elizabeth as charismatic and politically adroit, he commented that her speech to the Committee on Education was understated, hitting only the necessary features needed to impress legislators present at the hearing. Charles, described by Amos as a powerful and influential statesman and educator, was reported as having delivered the pivotal comment that solidified approval of the college. Charles was quoted in his declaration that Harvard decides once, it decides well, and it does not refute its decisions.

Amos reported that he was now authorized by his editor at *The Boston Daily Globe* to follow the "Radcliffe College story," a story, the editor had claimed, "that would surely evolve provocatively in this era of the women's movement." Universally pleased with Amos's article, the table turned toward Caroline.

Caroline recognized the unlikelihood of her appearance in Charles's office. Feeling out of place and outmatched, but pleased to be present, she described her new role to Charles.

"Ellen, my brother Stubby's wife, is very sick. She will be discharged from Waltham Hospital this week, returning home. Stubby and I will care for her." Caroline had promised Ellen that she would replace her at the Boston regional section of the General Federation of Women's Clubs. Reminding the group that Ellen was a strong advocate for women's education, and more generally, women's rights, Caroline pledged to support college education for nurses and a Harvard school of nursing.

"The Boston Women's Club stands with you on your next goal."

Looking directly at Annette, Caroline added, smiling, "I stand with you."

Mother and daughter smiled knowingly at each other. They were, finally, on the same side.

Rising from his chair, Charles stood, adjusted his glasses, and in rapid succession indicated specific areas for investigation regarding formation of a Harvard school of nursing. These areas included development of a budget and college infrastructure; management of opponents such as hospital administrators, doctors, and insurance companies; design of a college-level nursing curriculum; and knowledge of the status of state legislation and regulation of trained nurses.

"Opponents," announced Charles, "must convert to advocates or be neutralized."

"Hospitals will fight closure of training schools. Remember, greed is the elephant in the room." Stressing that the establishment of the school must follow a strategic path with well-formulated tactics, Charles intended to identify individuals to stage the battle.

He began with budget. "Money drives hospital administrators. Capitalism, as those who looked closely at the innovations showcased during the World's Fair last year saw, requires workers," Charles said, noting that "trained nurses are workers, basic hospital equipment."

"By increasing nurse training schools," he continued, "hospital income will increase, with more revenue for administrators and doctors. At the least, they will view our goal as a bothersome expense rather than a revenue source."

Charles stopped in front of Alistair and Millie.

"Millie and I will prepare a budget, investigate possible endowments, and design an administrative infrastructure for the school." Alistair, tapping his pen on his writing pad, seemed exceptionally eager to undertake this work. He reassured Charles that they had already begun this task.

"I am confident that we can achieve this," reassured Millie. "Alistair and I will begin our task now, reporting back at scheduled times. Annette and I graduate from Radcliffe this June, and, although I will then be assuming a teaching assistant position at the Cambridge School for Girls, I can be available in my free time for this project."

Nodding assent, Charles remained in front of Alfred.

"Alfred, you and I can negotiate with the clinical facilities we currently employ for student rotations at our medical school to expand rotations for nursing students. It'll be tricky. Some of them, such as Massachusetts General Hospital, operate nurse training schools. Will your colleagues at Waltham Hospital support our goal? Or will they be our opponents?" Alfred reported that board members of the Waltham Hospital had endorsed the gradual transition of their training school to a Harvard school of nursing. Perhaps Edward Cutler, Alfred offered, would join them in their visits.

Charles turned to Annette.

"Annette, you will continue to work with Alfred and Charlotte to design a four-year nursing curriculum, correct?" Charles spoke head down, peering over his eyeglasses. While assuring him that she would spearhead this effort, Annette noted that she would continue her master's degree in the classics after graduating with her bachelor's degree in two months.

"I intend to graduate with my AM degree in 1896," she said, assuring the room of the inevitable reality of the success she had always known.

They shared a glance, and an understanding.

Charles enlisted Alistair as his special envoy in the realm of legislation, including both nurse registration and regulation. Aware that the American Society of Superintendents of Training Schools for Nurses was recently established, at least in part to advocate for boards of examiners of nurses for the purpose of passing licensure regulations, Charles knew this matter to be of utmost importance. Licensure regulations are law. Harvard's medical school faculty were keeping a vigilant eye on actions related to the establishment of the Massachusetts Board of Registration in Medicine, an entity to license physicians and surgeons to practice in the state if they met registration requirements. In the case of medicine, the state legislature was expected to approve the bill in summer 1894. Charles and his crew needed to be fully versed in the status of nursing regulations and registration, similar to regulations in medicine.

"Alistair, consider drawing Charlotte into this work. Since she is a nursing school superintendent, she can be a valuable first lieutenant in ferreting information on the status of nurse registration." A shrewd banker, Alistair, ever charming and charismatic, would be capable of soliciting information easily, a trait that Charles believed invaluable in future conversation with legislators on the volatile subject of regulation and nurse registration. Charles was comfortable that, combined with Charlotte's insider knowledge of nurse leaders' thinking, Alistair and Alfred would devise workable tactics to secure the information they needed.

Charles then returned to the topic of opponents.

"Perhaps," he quipped, smiling, "we should begin with the easier question: *Who will support* a Harvard school of nursing?" Such needles in a haystack, Charles smirked, formed a short list. Over a working lunch of mince pies, plum pudding, and tea, the crew began to name people of influence, identifying them as advocates, opponents, or undecided. They completed their meeting and dispersed in the late March afternoon, the sky as clouded as when the day began.

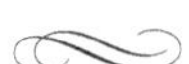

June 1894. I will soon be a Radcliffe College *Cliffie*, the informal name ascribed to Radcliffe students and graduates, Annette mused, curious if her life would change in any significant way after President Elizabeth Agassiz handed her a diploma and President Charles Eliot shook her hand.

Annette recalled the previous year's graduation account of Harvard Annex Class Day, held on Wednesday, June 21st, 1893, reported in *The Post*. Her father had written that the graduation was held as an "*en fete* event," with dancing, pretty girls, professors, crimson and white ribbons, lawns, laces, and fair seniors and juniors. As a member of the Idler Club, Annette, a junior at that time, had served as usher at that event. Seniors' guests were escorted into various lecture halls in Fay House that were transformed by flowers, light furniture, cushions, and colorful drapes into festive parlors. Japanese lanterns adorned the small campus, a soft glow permeating the outside atmosphere. Crimson and white the predominant colors. Following Class Day, formal commencement occurred in Sanders Theatre, also known as Memorial Hall, during a ceremony at which graduates received certificates signed by both Charles Eliot and Elizabeth Agassiz.

Annette winced at both the event itself and her father's reporting. The language spoke to her mother's world, not her own.

Great change, she thought, would be unlikely, and the lanterns and flowers would likely reappear at her Radcliffe graduation.

Annette would remain at the college to obtain her master's degree. She would then teach Greek and Latin at the Cambridge School for Girls, having already been promised a position by Arthur Gilman. At the Cambridge School, she would work with Millie, preparing promising young women for acceptance to Radcliffe College. As a known feeder program for Radcliffe, Gilman's school enjoyed elite status with a reputation as a sophisticated, highly respected enterprise among Back Bay residents. A position at the Cambridge School would be impressive.

She wondered if she should stay in that gilded cage or flee into a world she herself was creating.

Having completed her final examinations in Greek and Latin just one week earlier, Annette began to prepare her graduation packet at her desk by a window facing the family's spacious backyard.

As she worked, Caroline knocked on her bedroom door, asking to discuss upcoming family events with her.

Caroline had changed over the past year, and Annette recognized that her mother was becoming a different woman. As Ellen became increasingly infirm with tuberculosis, Caroline had assumed a role of assistant, a personal confidante. Now engaged in life beyond her kitchen, Caroline's participation in Charles's recent planning meeting was a sentinel moment in her mother's life. Imperceptibly, Ellen had segued Caroline into a key role in women's causes, serving as her replacement in the regional Women's Club in Boston. Embracing suffrage and education for women, Caroline no longer plagued Annette about bloomers, day dresses, cakes, or suitors. Had Ellen sneaked her mother a cigarette? Annette smiled to herself.

"Annie, I want to plan your graduation party, and a wedding dinner for Philip and Abigail. I want their wedding dinner first, although the wedding itself is not until July."

As she stood by Annette's desk, Caroline fidgeted with a ribbon on her day dress.

"I am sure that Abigail is pregnant, although neither she nor Philip have told me yet. I simply know from experience that this is true."

Shocking news to Caroline, but not so for Annette. After graduating from Harvard, Philip relocated to a new apartment in Cambridge, beginning his new life as a newspaper reporter, following his father's path. Confiding in Annette, Philip said that Abigail would also relocate to his apartment, indicating that they would marry by the end of the year. Pregnancy seemed inevitable to Annette. Understanding that a newspaper position, a pretty wife, and a young family were Philip's goals, Annette was pleased for him. With more space available in the family home, Annette was also pleased for herself, Millie, and Charlotte. Millie and Charlotte could occasionally spend the night in her brother's old room after a long day of outlining curricular plans for the nursing school.

"Mother, simply speak with Philip and Abigail about your suspicion. Once that is confirmed, I will help you plan a dinner for them and our two families. We will make it a lovely party and little else will matter." Annette buoyed Caroline's spirits, encouraging her mother to be joyful about a grandchild, rather than to be worried about what her neighbors might think of Abigail's out-of-wedlock pregnancy. Convincing her mother that one party was enough this summer, Annette sought to postpone her own graduation party until 1896, when she completed her graduate degree. Visibly relieved by Annette's offer, Caroline asked that she and Marguerite make their own arrangements with her dressmaker for wedding apparel.

Caroline lingered at her daughter's desk. "I enjoy the work I do with Ellen. It is stimulating, and time-consuming. Thank you, Annie, for helping me. I must say that contributing outside of my own home has been thrilling. I am beginning to understand, and appreciate, efforts made by women now." Caroline encircled her arms around her daughter, then left the room, saying she was off to the library on Ellen's behalf. With dressmaking and a graduation party off her calendar, Caroline left smiling.

Final examinations, marriage, pregnancy, parties, graduation, and dressmaking. I am awash with it all, thought Annette. Feelings of ambiguity, questioning, doubt, had begun to infiltrate Annette's quiet, intellectual life. Will teaching Greek and Latin be enough?

Surveying her bookshelves, Annette's eyes lingered on a large brown envelope containing Charles's 1869 articles in *The Atlantic*.

Gripping the envelope, Annette felt a growing, intense anger. What have I gained, and what have I lost, with Charles' new education?

Am I a young woman in a dying field? Annette wondered. Where will my knowledge get me, other than as a teacher in a classroom of girls? Dedicated to the establishment of a Harvard school of nursing, Annette wondered if she had become simply an instrument to accomplish the goals of others. Or was she integral to the enterprise? Was her background in logic and reasoning essential, or was she simply doing the bidding of influential men?

Annette completed her graduation packet, leaving home for Fay House. She knew that she must speak with Charles directly.

Alfred had been caught off guard. Alistair, Charlotte, and he had scheduled a meeting at the Waltham Training School reading room to explore current efforts to establish nurse registration and state regulations. Alistair, however, had come with an uninvited guest.

David Furst, Alistair's Chicago friend, was staying at the Campbells' home for a visit to Boston. Tall, thin, with thick brown hair cropped short and piercing brown eyes, David matched Alistair in charm, cordiality, and language. After introducing David as a graduate of Yale University's Law School, Alistair noted that David's legal practice involved dealings with Illinois's state regulations, including matters of health affairs.

"Since David's knowledge complements our need, he has offered to advise us as we tease out regulatory and registration matters in our own state."

"I'm pleased to be of assistance, should you have any questions I can address," said David, smiling, sipping the tea Charlotte gave him. Seated casually in a chair next to Charlotte at the conference table, David wrote the date in pencil on a small pad before him.

Now that Alfred knew more about the guest, he began the meeting with a summary of the Massachusetts Medical Society. "Perhaps," Alfred began, "a review of the society will help us understand the goals of the newly established American Society of Superintendents of Training Schools for Nurses."

The Medical Society, according to Alfred, was incorporated in 1781 for the purposes of advancing medical knowledge, developing and maintaining ethical standards for medical practice, and promoting medical institutions to benefit the welfare of citizens. Placing his Medical Society pamphlet on the table, Alfred noted that the state's organization was founded sixty-six years before the American Medical Association. Although the society at present did not oversee medical education, he stated that there was talk that it would soon develop a committee to accredit medical education programs.

"Doctors," Alfred offered, "worry that quacks might be licensed to practice. To prevent this, two actions are currently being promoted: the establishment of a board of registration in medicine and accreditation of medical education by the Medical Society."

An active alumnus of the Harvard Medical School, Alfred was knowledgeable of both intended actions. An act to establish the Massachusetts Board of Registration in Medicine was expected to be passed this June, according to Alfred. Since it had no significant opposition, the bill was expected to be approved by the legislature unanimously. Once the bill was passed, individuals graduating from a legally chartered medical college or university having power to confer degrees in medicine, plus anyone who has been a practitioner of medicine in the state continuously for a period of three years, would be entitled to registration and given a license to practice upon paying the required fee.

"The Medical Society," according to Alfred, "galvanized doctors to lobby for legislation creating a board of registration in medicine to register graduates of legally chartered medical programs to practice medicine."

Alistair and Charlotte immediately saw the parallels between medicine's and nursing's efforts. "Essentially," said Charlotte, "the newly established nursing society intends to follow the Medical Society's pattern. Secure nurse registration through legislation. I have been told that Mary Riddle, superintendent of Boston City Hospital, has approached Congressman Joseph H. Walker to sponsor a nursing registration bill. Lucy Drown and other nurse leaders are eager to learn Walker's reaction to Riddle's request."

David raised a finger at the group while jotting words on his pad. "May I," he asked, "take a few minutes to comment on medicine's registration board?" Annette and Millie both saw that, like Alistair, David's every gesture signaled relaxed confidence and keen intelligence.

"Nurse leaders cannot follow the medical registration board pattern for one major reason." Looking at Alfred, he asked when Harvard's Medical School was established. Alfred, patient with David's seemingly unrelated question, answered 1782. Continuing, David asked if Harvard was a legally chartered university with the authority to grant degrees in medicine. Without hesitation, Alfred responded that Harvard was founded by vote of the Great and General Court of Massachusetts in October of 1636, authorizing it to award degrees to graduates.

"How many legally chartered colleges and/or universities are currently authorized to award degrees in nursing?" David, looking at each of his hosts separately, knew the answer to his own question.

"None," Alfred and Charlotte answered concurrently.

"So, you see, nursing's registration board must differ from medicine's," said David. While much of the language in the bill creating the Board of Registration in Medicine could be easily modified for a board of registration of nurses, David encouraged the group to consider legal principles to guide their work.

"First, laws are dynamic; they are amended over time as conditions and context change." Continuing, David said that since nurses are now trained in schools owned by hospitals, medicine's language could easily be modified to accommodate this reality. The phrase "legally chartered colleges or universities with power to award degrees" might be replaced by "training schools owned by legally incorporated hospitals to provide nurse education," or, alternatively, applicants for nurse registration could be required to present a certificate or diploma attesting to completion of a training program. "Remember," David reminded, "laws evolve incrementally. Once colleges award degrees in nursing, then the initial law can be amended in this section."

"Second, there is a dearth of seasoned, senior nursing teachers. Doctors teach nurses today." David advised broad language in terms of training program structure, faculty, and clinical education. While a minimum educational program may be required, providing additional severe restrictions on numbers and types of patient experiences may be punitive, limiting the number of annual graduates. In one to two decades, David predicted, a pool of experienced, trained nurses may be available for instruction, particularly as hospital construction grows exponentially. And, he added, as more women enroll in colleges and are eventually granted the right to vote, nursing will surely transition to degree programs, similar to medicine and dentistry.

"Lastly, nursing care to individuals and families is currently provided by untrained nurses. Consider language that would allow them to register based on years of experience, without evidence of a diploma or certificate." David noted that this grandfather clause was occasionally used in laws approved in some southern states after the Civil War. He ended with a general reminder of the nature of these three legal principles.

"Laws provide a safety net against incompetent practitioners. Over time, laws may gradually become more stringent."

Again, silence as Alfred, Alistair, and Charlotte thought through David's comments.

Alistair, responding first, summarized his thoughts quite generically. "Under David's framework, we would do well to focus on the power held by elected legislators. The more we consider why legislation has evolved the way that it has, the better our chance of success."

"You have captured it well, Alistair," smiled David. "Crafting legislation that enables the registration of trained nurses while not threatening wealthy, powerful men orchestrating hospital expansion will require cunning politics on your side," he added.

"David, there is another problem to explore," added Charlotte. "Nurse leaders view trained nurses as hospital tools. I believe leaders will demand registration be granted only to trainees having specific years of experience in hospitals offering certain services and bed capacity. They will not be on the side of reasonable legislation awarding registration certificates to applicants having different experiences from their demands. These leaders will be our enemies."

"At present," Charlotte added, "nurse leaders do not endorse suffrage efforts. They do not support women, neither voting rights nor education."

David leaned forward in his chair, intent to refocus the group on practical, political strategies to achieve their goals. He fired off multiple questions in rapid succession.

"Since these agendas are at play, as they always are in legislation, then you must be sharply focused on how to garner support for reasonable, broad legislation. What powerful legislators will support you? Have any of you supported legislators to help pass specific bills? Does any legislator owe you support? What powerful men might be on your side? Are there any wealthy donors supportive of your cause for a Harvard school of nursing? Since hospital administrators are now organizing, what are your relationships with any of these individuals? What is in it for the powerful legislators, men, and hospital capitalists that Alistair spoke of previously?" David stopped, realizing that he had pivoted the discussion to a political campaign, a twist that the group had not anticipated.

"If the very nurse leaders you wish to support via broad legislation may be your enemies, then you will need political warriors on your team. It may be time to put on helmets, raise your shields, and build an army of supportive legislators and other powerful men. Wage war, if you are wedded to the importance of your cause." Rising from his chair, David stretched and raised his teacup to Alfred, Alistair, and Charlotte.

"You came. You saw. You will succeed."

After thanking David for his insights, Alfred invited the group, including David, if his time permitted, to meet in one week to map out a campaign to garner support for a non-restrictive board of registration of nurses, reasonable requirements for nurse registration, and the establishment of a Harvard school of nursing. While he knew of Moses T. Stevens and William Shadrach Knox, Massachusetts legislators in the US House of Representatives from District Five, including Waltham and most of Cambridge, Alfred admitted that he had little knowledge of their political stance on current major issues. While Stevens had not completed his degree at Dartmouth College, he was well regarded as a shrewd politician, businessman, and bank president. Knox, a Republican, would succeed Stevens. A graduate from Amherst College in law, Knox had served as city solicitor in Lawrence for several years before becoming, like Stevens, a bank president.

"We must meet our district representatives. Become familiar with their political leanings. We must influence them. Perhaps they may introduce a bill along the lines David has suggested." Alfred asked Annette and Alistair if they would join him in introductory meetings with Stevens and Knox. Both agreed, with David stating that he would also join them if his schedule permitted.

"This has been a productive meeting," Alfred concluded as he promised to review Stevens's voting record and other relevant information prior to scheduling meetings.

"Developing relationships is critical," said David, as he shook hands with Alfred and Alistair, and patted Charlotte's back. "Win them to your side."

As Alfred left the training school, he contemplated one more twist. Should they focus first on the establishment of the Harvard School of Nursing, or spend time on the wording of regulations for nurse registration in the state? Both were important, but which would carry the most political sway?

Early for her appointment to speak with Charles Eliot, Annette waited in his office, wavering in her resolve. Wearing a dark-blue, full-length A-line skirt complemented by a white blouse with high collar and narrow sleeves, Annette was fashionably attired. Her mother had been quite satisfied. But, she wondered, perhaps even her dress had become part of the problem. Had she been too willing to please and, as a result, become little more than a tool for others? And, in that process, had she been complicit in devaluing a field of study she had come to love?

"Annette, a pleasure to see you again. Still working on the nursing curriculum?" Ever charming, Charles smiled.

With his eyeglass frame circling tightly around each ear, snarling graying hair untidily at his neck, Charles was unusually buoyant and uncharacteristically talkative.

"Lizzie and I look forward to your graduation in a few days," Charles said, now sitting at his desk, rifling quickly through his mail folder as if searching for something specific.

"Ah, here it is!"

Charles opened the large brown envelope carefully and slowly, with reverence. Gently, he removed a single paper from the envelope, holding it up for Annette to see. It was a picture of the Radcliffe arms, symbolizing Lady Ann Moulshan's maiden Radcliffe family coat of arms.

"This is Radcliffe College's shield, recognizing Ann Moulshan's gift of one hundred pounds to Harvard College in 1643. This gift was placed in a new fund, the Lady Moulshan Scholarship

Fund established last year, the first such gift given to a college by a woman. The fund will be used in support of Radcliffe College students." Charles, visibly pleased with himself, returned the picture to its envelope, placing it on the top of his mail pile.

Returning to Annette, Charles asked for the purpose of her visit. "Nursing efforts, I presume?"

"No, my reasons for seeing you go deeper," Annette spoke clearly, evenly, looking directly at Charles.

"Twenty-five years ago, you advocated a new system of education for America. One based on pure and applied sciences, living European languages, and mathematics, instead of upon Greek, Latin, and mathematics. Such a system now exists at Harvard, for men. I, however, will receive my undergraduate degree in the classics this month, and my master's degree in the same in two years."

Annette paused.

"What was your rationale for advancing the changes you introduced during your first years as president, and when will women enjoy the broader degree options available to men?" Unsure if she had been clear, Annette started to speak again when Charles interrupted.

"I understand your questions. It appears that you want to see if I have ever reflected on my inaugural address. And you want to see how my changes will result in broader change."

Annette knew why she wavered before entering the office of someone who understood everything in an instant.

"Your first question is an easy one to answer. We learned how ignorant we were as a country as the Civil War waged on for years. We quickly learned that our need for ministers must be complemented by scientists in engineering, medicine, mining, and other fields, fields that depended on knowledge from basic and applied sciences. And, since educational resources are, in fact, limited and oftentimes dependent on endowments, we needed to decrease some courses in order to offer new ones if we hoped to balance our books." Charles, Annette realized, did not hesitate to shift resources to advance technological progress. He was remorseless.

"It was a very simple matter, Annette. There was, and still is, no question about the need for science. I shifted course emphasis once, and I would do it again without blinking."

"Your second question is complex." Walking toward the large window facing a lush garden, Charles took his time answering Annette. "You want to know how long it will take for everyone to be lifted by the tide of my actions."

"Women do not yet enjoy the same status as men in America. They do not vote, although I suspect that will change soon. Annette, your experiences have been different from most women in America. You are a Back Bay resident educated first at the Gilman's Cambridge School and now at Radcliffe College. While your college course choices have not included medicine or basic sciences, you are sagacious and appreciate that gains for women will be incremental. First, college education, then voting rights, then employment opportunities. Changes in our society, our culture, will follow."

"Do not ignore the current context. Nursing is a valuable option for women now. Health care is opening to you, providing employment and opportunities to contribute to society beyond marriage and motherhood. Women can capture and expand these opportunities, creating rapid change, shaping our country's future."

Charles faced Annette.

"I have done my part, and now it is up to you to lift yourself. Do you wish to be a nurse?"

Annette added firmly, "I want my master's degree, and I wish to be a nurse."

"Then you have answered your own questions," Charles replied as he returned to his desk. "You will complete your education in the profession you have loved your entire life, and you will begin a profession you have begun to love to ensure that you will be lifted up."

He tugged a little on the hair on the back of his neck, adjusted his glasses, and smiled.

Signaling that the meeting had ended, Charles walked Annette to the door.

"I am wagering on you, as a new nurse leader, to turn our country's focus to health, to a public system of preventive care. I have taken risks and gambled in my past. I have never lost."

Smiling, Charles shook Annette's hand and led her out of his office.

Annette walked home briskly, despite the warm weather. She saw her future clearly.

She would have both, at their best.

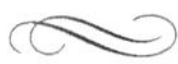

Against a cloudless, sunny June day, President Elizabeth Agassiz and President Charles W. Eliot sat together on the stage of Harvard's Sanders Theatre, a building with capacity for one thousand occupants and renowned for its acoustics. Completed in 1875, the theatre was routinely used for commencements, concerts, ceremonies, and professional conferences.

On this day, the Radcliffe College Class of 1894 was the first to receive Radcliffe degrees. Framed against brilliant crimson and white banners hanging from the ceiling and classical Tuscany urns filled with bouquets of pungently aromatic spring tulips and red roses lining the walls, twenty-two graduates received baccalaureate degrees signed by both Radcliffe College and Harvard University presidents. Family, friends, and faculty participated in the commencement exercises, followed by a late luncheon hosted by Alice Mary Longfellow in her home on Brattle Street.

Presidents Agassiz and Eliot congratulated Annette and Millie as they received their diplomas. Immediately after the graduation ceremony, Annette and Millie discarded their academic regalia of black gowns with crow's feet emblems near the yoke and donned festive white and crimson day dresses given to them as gifts from Caroline and Amos.

Annette, Alfred, Millie, and Alistair toasted their victory, drinking champagne in the Longfellow Garden.

"Perhaps," Annette whispered to Millie, "we can steal away for a few minutes. I have cigarettes stashed in my dress pocket." Laughing, Millie joined Annette as Alfred and Alistair mingled with other guests in the parlor.

Enjoying warm breezes while on swings in the garden, they delighted in silence and cigarettes. Eventually, Millie spoke of her own imminent future. She looked forward to serving as an assistant teacher at Gilman's Cambridge School for Girls. Annette said that she would remain a student of Greek and Latin at Radcliffe, then dropped her bombshell.

"Millie, I must tell you that I want to become a nurse, perhaps training at the Waltham School after obtaining my master's degree if the Harvard School of Nursing is not established in two years."

Millie, incredulous, with eyes wide open, was about to speak when Caroline ran over to them in the garden. She held her daughter close.

"It's Ellen. She's dead."

Accomplishment

"Once again, as I have just said, I strongly suggest that you speak with Mary Riddle, the superintendent of the Boston City Hospital. She has already fully versed us regarding licensure of trained nurses."

Dabbing sweat from his forehead, John Roberts, the thin, young, bespectacled legal assistant for Congressman Joseph H. Walker, rose so abruptly from his desk that his chair noisily tumbled backward to the floor. He was becoming increasingly flabbergasted at the insistent young woman standing on the other side of his desk, flanked by two bemused men.

Believing that more detail might persuade these stubborn people to go away, Roberts described recent discussions with Mary Riddle and several of her colleagues. Riddle, currently assistant superintendent of nurses at Boston City Hospital, was leading a campaign to legislate the establishment of a board of registration of nurses that would register trained nurses, thus, differentiating untrained nurses from trained nurses. The effort was similar to planning for a board of registration in medicine. Roberts indicated that Riddle and her colleagues hoped to emulate the medical board to establish a similar one for nursing.

As Roberts struggled to maintain his composure, Annette said that perhaps it would be best to simply go to the congressman's office. Alistair and David grinned at hearing that withering tone, surely borrowed from Millie. Annette spun to walk toward the door.

As Roberts gestured to prevent Annette barging into his boss's office, a stack of papers teetering precariously on his desk began to fall to the floor. Annette turned back to catch them just in time. Their eyes met, Annette smiled, and he smiled back. Alistair and David knew that Roberts had been defeated.

"Mr. Roberts, may we begin again?" Annette asked slowly, calmly, in a drawing room voice that might have been that of her mother.

As would an obedient dog, Roberts sat.

"Please accept my apologies. While my morning thus far has been a bit disastrous, I regret that I have displaced my frustration on you. Yes, please let us begin again." Smiling, Roberts shook hands with Annette, Alistair, and David. Checking the congressman's calendar, he saw that, indeed, an appointment had been made and that his efforts to redirect this woman and her companions had been misplaced. He began to provide useful information, beginning with the concept of registration.

"The medical board became fully effective on January 1st of this year," Roberts added, while noting that there were key differences between the language of the medical board and the proposed language of the nurse's bill regarding requirements for registration.

"Tell us more," said David, ever the attorney. "How do the proposed requirements for nursing registration differ from those in medicine?" Leaning on Roberts's desk, pen in hand and eyes riveted on the legal assistant, David's intensity encouraged deep engagement in the topic. Although Charles had enlisted Alistair as his special legislative envoy, Alistair was glad he had brought David with him to the meeting, along with Annette. Each had unique talents that would be invaluable in legal matters that Charles knew to be of the utmost importance.

Thumbing through Section Three of the Board of Registration in Medicine Act, Roberts read to David that "graduates of a legally chartered medical college or university having power to confer degrees in medicine, and every person who has been a practitioner of medicine in this commonwealth continuously for a period of three years next prior to the passage hereof, shall upon the payment of a fee of one dollar be entitled to registration and the board shall issue him a certificate." Additionally, he noted that any person not entitled to registration according to the requirements above was entitled to examination and if found qualified, would be registered as a physician.

"By comparison, while doctors link registration to college or university degrees, nurses want registration tied to training in hospitals." Roberts continued, reading the language crafted by Riddle and her colleagues to be embedded in a bill to be sponsored by Walters. He then read from Section Three of the bill:

"Applicants for registration shall satisfy said board by presentation of diploma or certificate, that he or she is a graduate of a training school for nursing giving at least a two years' course, or a proper equivalent for a part thereof, in the theory and practice of nursing in a hospital, or shall present a certificate from a general hospital giving evidence of a two years' course of training in the theory and practice of nursing, or certificates from one or more hospitals, general or special, giving evidence of having pursued at least a two years' course of training in the theory and practice of nursing in a hospital."

And, similar to medicine, he added that nurse leaders sought examinations as part of the registration procedure.

"What does Congressman Walker think of Riddle's proposed nursing bill?" asked Alistair.

Roberts began with a standard response. "Joseph Walker is intent to help the nurses, along with all his constituencies, achieve their goals." Roberts then lowered his voice, taken with the earnestness of those standing across from him.

"Walker has a problem with the nurses' proposed bill."

"What problem?" asked Alistair as Annette stepped closer to Roberts's desk.

"Their bill stands against education. Walker advocates for education, not apprenticeships, not preceptorships." Roberts reminded them that while Walker's background prior to politics was exclusively in the business of manufacturing leather goods, his son, also named Joseph, had earned degrees from Brown University, Harvard College, and Harvard Law School. He was particularly proud of his son's admittance to the Suffolk County bar in 1889.

"Nurses, according to both father and son," claimed Roberts, "must be educated, as are doctors, dentists, lawyers, engineers, and others. Education and suffrage are particular passions of Walker's son. On occasion, however, my boss will fall back on tradition. He is, after all, a politician and needs every vote." Roberts indicated that he was personally campaigning with the younger Walker to dissuade his father from this distinction.

"So, you see, Congressman Walker will, no doubt, continue to work with Mary Riddle and her colleagues. And I will continue to help him recognize that there is something else at play here, something almost dark, abhorrent."

Drawn in by Roberts's last statement, Annette asked that he expand on his thoughts. What abhorrent thing permeated Riddle's cause?

Although saying that it was difficult to put a name to it, Roberts claimed that Riddle's tenacious grip on hospital-based training to the exclusion of other forms of education was an overwhelming blind spot in current nurse leaders' thinking.

"These women are being manipulated by hospitals." Sharing that his sister was a pupil nurse at a local hospital training school, Roberts was appalled by her reports of exhaustion, intermittent coursework, and overwhelming domestic tasks.

Their discussion over, Roberts led them quietly through the dimly lit Honduras mahogany wood-paneled halls toward Walker's office. Annette glanced into the House chamber, circular in configuration, noting the four-foot, eleven-inch Sacred Cod hanging over the public gallery, symbolizing the importance of the fishing industry within the state. The plate on Walker's door was gold, with his name in dark letters: Joseph H. Walker. As Elizabeth Agassiz had felt months earlier during the Committee on Education's hearing to award Radcliffe College degree-granting authority, Annette was impressed into silence, almost reverence.

These men have the power to change lives, she thought. Women, however, did not yet have the right to vote. Why would any legislator sponsor a bill for a constituency who cannot vote? Such a bill may not only waste time, but also incur the wrath of powerful men.

Annette had begun to see behind the curtain.

With a shock of wavy, snow-white hair cropped short and sporting dense, grayish-white muttonchop sideburns, Joseph Henry Walker surprised Charles's crew by opening his door wide and welcoming them to his office with his deep baritone voice.

"Come in! Do come in." Gesturing for them to take seats in armchairs framing his desk in a broad semicircle, Walker returned to his faded dark-brown leather padded chair, which comfortably accommodated his large frame.

Smiling, he asked simply, "Why are you here today? How can I help you? As I understand it from my calendar, your appointment concerns nursing education."

Pleased by Walker's affable welcome, yet somewhat dubious of his friendliness, David reviewed their previous conversation with his legal assistant, John Roberts. Could Walker kindly update them on his legislative efforts with Mary Riddle? Unsure as to how much detail from their conversation with Roberts was appropriate to share, David largely focused on the main difference between the proposed requirements for nurse registration and those now in effect for physician registration.

"The primary difference between the requirements might be simply stated," Alistair added. "Collegiate education for doctors versus apprenticeship training for nurses."

"Ah," said Walker, shaking his head purposively.

"Wait here for a moment." Walker left the room, only to return a few minutes later with a younger man at his side.

"Let me introduce my son, Joseph," said the older man proudly. The younger Joseph shook hands with his father's guests, looking quite uncomfortable as his father bragged about the accomplishments of his son.

Tall and thin, with hair slicked back by Macassar oil and wearing gold-rimmed Windsor glasses, the younger Joseph was stern, quite unlike his engaging father. As he sat, he took care to avoid leaning his oiled hair against the chair's backrest.

After a brief silence, Alistair spoke first, noting that he, his two companions, and perhaps Joseph appeared to have several interests in common, among them college education and law. Both Joseph and he were Harvard graduates, Annette held a Radcliffe College degree, and David was a Yale law graduate. After a brief, friendly verbal tussle over the merits of Harvard versus Yale law, the younger Joseph, serving only as advisor to his father, extended their mutual interests to the subject before them, nursing education, and what he described as its "horrifying shortcomings."

In agreement that changes were needed to the bill's language, yet dissenting from his son's characterization, Congressman Walker said that he represented District Three in the current fifty-third congress, which included twenty-six towns in Middlesex and Worcester Counties. Previously, he had represented District Ten, but due to population shifts noted in the 1890 US census, he now represented more residents in a broader, neighboring area. Given that his guests were represented by congressmen in other districts, he suggested they widen their lobbying to include representatives from Districts Eight and Four. He proposed that a nursing registration bill could be co-sponsored by Samuel McCall, District Eight, which included Cambridge, and Lewis Apsley, District Four, which included Waltham.

"A co-sponsored bill is more likely to be approved than one with a single sponsor," the congressman suggested, winking at them. Glancing at his son and David, he assured them that McCall was a seasoned Massachusetts lawyer and that Apsley, founder of a rubber clothing company, was a shrewd entrepreneur and statesman. In fact, he had already sent McCall a note about their mutual interest in nursing licensure. Given redistricting, and upon Walker's advice, Alistair agreed to concentrate on McCall and Apsley as co-sponsors with Walker on legislative efforts, rather than on Stevens or Knox.

Walker advised them to see if McCall might speak with them today. David and the younger Joseph agreed to draft revised language for what they now termed the Riddle Bill. Once McCall and Apsley came on board as co-sponsors, Congressman Walker would invite Mary Riddle and her colleagues to discuss any revised language and the rationale for the suggested changes.

"You might remind these representatives that the suffrage movement is a powerful one, rumbling down the road toward us. New voters. All congressmen would do well to advocate for women's causes, their education, and welfare."

Shaking each of their hands with both of his, Walker led them graciously from his office.

Annette realized that she had been wrong. While a constituency of women could not yet vote, legislators had realized that the time for change was upon them.

Annette, Alistair, and David felt heard.

Sitting in a sturdy wooden churchlike pew outside Samuel McCall's office, Alistair, David, and Annette were thankful that the congressman was available to see them without advance scheduling. No doubt, thought David, their meeting would be a favor to his colleague, Congressman Walker.

"Politicians understand colleagueship, the building of relationships. As long as favors do not run to corruption, I certainly appreciate congressmen aligning on important issues," said David. Annette and Alistair were somewhat surprised that he had spoken aloud his feelings on the fluid border between politics and self-interest.

Alistair, raising an eyebrow at David, asked if he recalled Charles Parkhurst, the Presbyterian minister born in Massachusetts who served as pastor at the Madison Square Presbyterian Church in New York City. A social reformer, Parkhurst had challenged Tammany Hall, advertised as a social club, only three years earlier, claiming it a society for politicians that, in Parkhurst's words "shields and patronizes iniquity; while we try to convert criminals, they manufacture them." Given progressives' current mandates for social reform and elimination of political corruption, Alistair advised that neutrality on politicians' behaviors was a wise position to assume. David nodded, appreciating his younger colleague's advice.

Sprinting toward them from the north end of the corridor, a young, well-dressed man waved at them, smiling broadly. Pushing thick, wavy dark-brown hair from his deep-blue eyes, he stopped in front of them, slightly bent over with hands on knees, chuckling that he needed just one moment to catch his breath. Annette smiled back, taken by his spontaneity and energy.

Standing to face him, Annette introduced herself, Alistair, and David. She glanced at his hands as he reached for hers, a three-second assessment she had learned to make. He did not wear a ring. Entering Congressman McCall's office, Alistair winked at

Annette. Staring back at him as her face blushed slightly, Annette sat in one of the chairs facing the congressman's desk.

"My name is Martin Byrne, Congressman Samuel McCall's legal assistant. It is a pleasure to meet you all." As Byrne left the office to tell the congressman that his visitors had arrived, Alistair whispered that either she got to know Byrne or he and David would. Scowling at Alistair, Annette hoped that McCall would enter soon and save her from these schoolboy antics.

Samuel McCall contrasted sharply with Walker. With a lean face and sharp, angular nose, McCall was balding, with closely cropped graying hair and prominent jutting chin. His tall, thin frame was impeccably clothed in a black suit and white shirt with starched wing collar. His stride was sure-footed, matching his patrician appearance and confidence. McCall conveyed seriousness, a no-nonsense politician who attended the New Hampton Literary and Biblical Institute and held an AB degree from Dartmouth College. After graduating, McCall studied law, gaining admission to the Massachusetts bar.

"Tell me about your interest in licensure for nurses and a board of registration for nurses, similar to what exists in medicine." McCall was all business.

"There is a tricky aspect to this bill, Congressman McCall," David began. He then provided background to the bill, describing Mary Margaret Riddle, the newly established American Society for Superintendents of Training Schools for Nurses, and the push for nurse training to be provided in hospitals, inferring control by hospital administrators for economic gain.

"Who supports nurse education in colleges?" asked McCall, shifting from opponents to advocates.

Annette responded. "President Eliot is eager to establish a Harvard school of nursing to complement the medical and dental schools. The proposal for a school has the endorsement of the Harvard Corporation and Board of Overseers."

"Good that Eliot is a strong advocate," replied McCall, delighted at the young woman's sense of referred clout.

"Bills, however, are always tricky, just as David says, resplendent with advocates and opponents. Bills are testaments to negotiation and compromise. We must get all parties to come together on one basic need — in this case, licensure of nurses — and then we'll negotiate on thorny details, knowing that most bills are amended over time as conditions warrant." McCall added he would appeal to Lewis Apsley, a rubber company entrepreneur, his newly elected colleague from District Four, to join Walker and him on a co-sponsored nurse bill.

Annette was pleased when the congressman asked Martin to take the lead on this bill. McCall also suggested meeting with President Eliot, noting that Martin was a Harvard-trained lawyer. This Harvard-oriented group, he noted, could have deep reach as far as legislation goes. Especially now, he chuckled, since Eliot's Harvardization of American colleges continued to sweep through the country.

Smiling assuredly, David complimented Annette and Alistair as they left the congressman's office and boarded the hansom cab to return to Cambridge. Grateful for David's kind words, Annette remained edgy about the legislative future in a world so often set against women. Yet Annette had watched her mother gravitate from her kitchen to meetings of the General Federation of Women's Clubs, largely due to exposure to Ellen. Change was possible.

She could still see her beloved aunt mimicking a long drag on an imaginary cigarette. She wished she were still with her so they could steal away to the gazebo and plan the future together.

Fortunately, Annette reflected, her graduate studies at Radcliffe were not overly burdensome. She always knew she would succeed before she began, and quiet translation remained a pleasurable interruption to her public work with Charles and the crew. She had come to realize that Charles was absolutely correct: establishing a Harvard school of nursing was much more time-consuming and politically fraught than obtaining degree-granting authority for Radcliffe College.

Enjoying sweetened peach tea in her family's garden with Millie and Alistair on a summer afternoon, Annette methodically reviewed actions taken toward establishing the Harvard School of Nursing.

"Well," said Millie, "we have completed a draft nursing curriculum, as well as identifying hospitals and other facilities — industrial sites, baby stations, and others — for student clinical rotations." Since it was too early to secure contracts for nursing student experiences at these facilities, Millie noted that Alfred and Charles would solidify such agreements as a final step in the process of incorporating the school. Additionally, legislative efforts toward licensure for nurses had already begun, with congressmen targeted to co-sponsor a bill as support mounted.

"We do not have endowments for the school yet, but . . ." Alistair grinned, not completing his sentence. He enjoyed the drama. Describing recent conversations with his father, Alistair indicated that he was willing to consider changing his planned Harvard endowment from the arts to the new school of nursing, pending one condition. Alistair then relayed his recent conversation with his father.

"As a businessman and a member of the Harvard Board of Overseers," Matthew Campbell had said to his son, "I want to see others also support the new school. Health is good business. I cannot be the single endowment. You must secure at least one other." Claiming that a single endowment from a board member would appear incestuous, Matthew challenged his son to attract other donors, perhaps one from beyond Back Bay.

"Perhaps," Matthew offered, "you might consider talking with Jacob H. Schiff."

"Schiff?" Alistair questioned, quizzical look on this face.

Matthew had been surprised that Alistair did not recognize Schiff's name. A New York City Jewish-American banker and businessman, Schiff had amassed a fortune through a variety of ventures, most prominently the expansion of American railroads. Incentivized by the Jewish principle of *Tzedakah*, an ethical obligation toward charity that bent that arc of humanity toward justice, and driven by his infuriation over antisemitism and sickness, Schiff supported diverse charitable endeavors with the aim of advancing his community.

"Alistair," his father continued, "Schiff has already given to Harvard. In January, 1890, he donated ten thousand dollars to Harvard for the creation of a museum dedicated to the literature, history, and remains of the Semitic peoples. *The New York Times* had a nice article about this, if you have time to review it."

Embarrassed that he had not recalled ongoing construction of a building on the Harvard campus designated for Semitic studies, Alistair thanked his father for his generous assistance.

Alistair then concluded the story of his conversation with a flourish: "We do not have endowments for the school yet, but we may have success with Schiff."

Hearing the name for a second time, Millie had jumped up, tumbling her peach tea onto a flowering bush.

"I have an idea!" she exclaimed, cheeks glowing, red with excitement.

"We need to visit Lillian Wald again." Millie continued, recalling that public health activities on the Lower East Side of Manhattan were supported by the same Jacob Schiff that Matthew's father praised so highly. Lillian's Henry Street settlement survived, in fact, thrived, she contended, with Schiff's support.

Alistair smiled.

"Yes, our draft curriculum might be of interest to Schiff," said Annette pensively. Yet she wondered if his support would extend to a nursing curriculum focusing on health education to others than the Jewish community in the Lower East Side of Manhattan.

"Because he is a Jewish American," Alistair responded, "I would imagine that Schiff understands the complexities of being *the other*. I too understand such complexities. It is difficult, if not impossible, to be blind to prejudice once you yourself have been victimized by it." Alistair offered to learn about Schiff, his charities, and especially, his support of health care efforts.

Annette offered to make arrangements for a visit to Lillian, noting that she would seek her counsel as to a meeting with Schiff to review Harvard's plan for a school of nursing.

Seeing an opportunity to advance their legislative efforts simultaneously with a visit to Wald and Schiff, Annette cleared her throat and asked Millie and Alistair if it might be wise to bring

Congressman McCall's legislative assistant with them to New York.

"If Martin Byrne were to join us," she offered, "he would immediately recognize the value of community and public health nursing. Nurse leaders' current mandate for two consecutive years of hospital training as a requirement for nurse licensure would appear ludicrous to him once he saw all that Lillian does." Annette kept her gaze on Millie, aware that Alistair was smiling broadly, clapping softly in response to her suggestion.

"Indeed!" exclaimed Millie. "We can broaden our crew, include a legislative aide as an advisor. If Congressman McCall will be a co-sponsor on the Walker bill, then by all means get Martin on board." Millie was proud of her friend's growing tactical ability. Caesar, she smiled to herself, would be proud.

Annette quietly enjoyed her two years of graduate studies, even as she worked with her crewmates on the Harvard curriculum. Now, as the Spring 1896 semester bloomed lavishly on the Radcliffe College campus, Annette skillfully managed several fronts concurrently. At home, Caroline celebrated Philip and Abigail's wedding, as well as the birth of their son Richard, in a lavish event in late March. To Annette's surprise, Caroline, who enjoyed her grandson, remained active as a full-time officer of the Boston regional section of the General Federation of Women's Clubs. She and Amos recruited a domestic kitchen maid for cleaning and meal preparation, thus relieving Caroline of major household responsibilities. For his part, Amos published feature article after feature article on women's education and the need for a Harvard school of nursing. And, after Ellen's death, Caroline's brother Stubby returned to his active faculty role at Harvard, with his adult children occasionally visiting for company.

Caroline and Stubby became again the brother and sister companions of their childhood. Frequently working together to organize women's events at his home, they became passionate about women's education, suffrage, and equal rights. Marguerite, Annette's sister, often provided musical entertainment, sometimes accompanied by Elizabeth, Alfred's wife. A musical duet, Marguerite and Elizabeth added elegance to what were sometimes contentious meetings over just how equal equal rights must be. Unlike the mother of Annette's childhood, Caroline was fueled by disagreements between youthful supporters of equal rights and opinionated older women who sometimes looked askance at brash proposals of equity. All of these events were attended by Amos, ready to publish on short notice.

Annette enjoyed it all. This stimulating environment thrilled her, encouraging creation of change.

At the last meeting of the crew in Charles's office, the addition of Martin Byrne as a political advisor was applauded, as well as the visit to Lillian Wald in New York City. Since Schiff had personally awarded Charles the gift to establish a Semitic museum at Harvard, Charles said that he would compose a letter requesting that he and Alfred meet with Schiff at Harvard House in New York City to describe plans for a school of nursing with a strong scientific and humanistic curriculum, including a focus on maintenance of health. The following day, Charles planned to meet Lillian Wald at the Henry Street Settlement with Alfred, Annette, and Charlotte.

"Jacob is practical. He will want to know the purpose of our visit." Charles indicated that he would write to him with a direct request to consider awarding seed funding to support some aspect of the school's infrastructure, possibly classrooms, library resources, faculty, or other pragmatic concerns. One must be cautious, Charles had advised, to be appropriate in any such request, particularly from previous donors.

"Annette, you have already met Schiff. Take time to learn everything you can about him." Charles encouraged them to explore what Judaism might mean to Schiff. How did his religious orientation impact his giving? What other charitable causes has he funded?

"Most importantly, learn as much as you can about the Henry Street Settlement. What does this settlement mean to him? Why does he support Lillian Wald?"

Charles concluded the meeting with a rare statement of gratitude.

"We have been working on our goals for several years now. We have achieved much in a very short time. Huzzah to each of you! Be patient. Perhaps in 1900 we will celebrate the first convocation at the Harvard School of Nursing. The start of our school is but a few years away." Raising his cup of tea, Charles nodded at the group, praising them with a genuine, heartfelt smile.

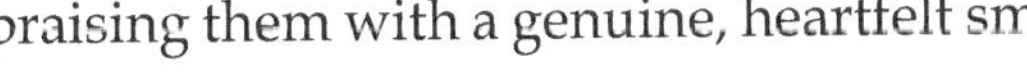

Once home, Annette sat at her desk in her room, anxious to organize her work for the remainder of her final graduate semester at Radcliffe. Comfortably cross-legged on the floor, with notepad and books arranged in a semicircle around her, Millie also worked, developing her next week's teaching plan for students at the Cambridge School for Girls. A teaching assistant, Millie viewed her work as neither challenging nor stimulating. The position, however, provided her secure space for her efforts as a member of Charles's crew. At the last meeting, Charles had invited her to consider a new role as an administrative assistant to the president on matters related to the proposed school of nursing. Once the school was approved by the legislature, she could then transfer to nursing as an administrator in the dean's office. Millie agreed immediately to Charles's offer, noting that she would begin her new duties when the school year ended at the Cambridge School.

I will keep my intellectual standing, thought Millie with pride.

Radicalized, Annette and Millie found their lives centered on the planned school of nursing and the liberation it represented. Millie frequently stayed in Philip's former bedroom to strategize and expedite plans. Their future was tangible, and they were almost there.

Annette, mind wandering, gazed out her window, reciting the first quatrain of Emily Dickinson's poem "Nobody Knows this Little Rose":

> *Nobody knows this little rose;*
> *It might a pilgrim be,*
> *Did I not take it from the ways,*
> *And lift it up to thee!*

The lines were comforting to hear, a recollection of something small, a gesture that would endure.

Annette spoke first, ending the silence between them. "I will invite Martin to join Elizabeth and me some weekend in April. Some real-life experiences will ground him in the broader health-oriented work of nurses in communities." Since their visits with Lillian Wald on Manhattan's Lower East Side were planned for late spring, Annette knew she had adequate time to introduce Martin to public health and community nursing in April. Some exposure was in order, she felt. With calendar in hand, Annette drew up a short clinical rotation of patient experiences for Martin, capitalizing on her visits to the milk stations and the baby unit within Waltham Hospital. Annette and Elizabeth Worcester provided volunteer services at these facilities on weekends, providing much needed care for children and young mothers in the city. The rotation would be a gesture, something important to her, and she wondered if he would see it as that or as an obligation to be met.

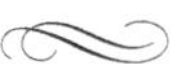

"A legislative aide, a lawyer visiting our milk stations? Our baby unit at Waltham Hospital?" Alfred was wary when Annette told him of her plan on a visit to his home. "How will Martin understand what he sees? It is not his world."

Annette nevertheless stressed exposure to health care and relationship-building as key ingredients to achieving their goal. Alfred could not hear Annette, choosing to concentrate on his suspicions about legislators instead.

Alfred's leeriness was overcome by his wife's excitement at having a legislative visitor accompany them on their weekend rounds.

"This will be marvelous, Alfred! He will see, firsthand, the needs of residents in his district. He can then advise the Congressman on actions to be taken. Thank you, Annette. I truly look forward to working with Martin and you next weekend." Energized, Elizabeth offered to pack lunch for them. Her mind raced about future fundraising musical events that she and Marguerite Fiske could organize.

A few days later, Martin enthusiastically agreed to participate at several milk stations in Waltham and to assist in an afternoon at the baby unit in Waltham Hospital. Alfred was quietly grateful that Martin would visit sick babies at the hospital, since baby care in the city was woefully inadequate, oftentimes fraught with infectious diseases difficult to contain. Alfred's goal was the establishment of a Waltham baby hospital, contiguous with, but independent from, the Waltham Hospital.

When he learned of the visit, Alfred begrudgingly realized that perhaps Annette was correct. Maybe relationship-building might prove fruitful. He smiled to himself when he thought of his wife's enthusiasm, her hope for a new world, and realized just how right Annette had been about so much on that snowy winter day.

"This is the first I have heard of milk stations," said Martin, squinting against the sunlight streaming on his face. What are these stations, he wondered, and how is nurse legislation related to this work? In fact, other than the chance to be in the company of a charming young woman, why am I here in the first place?

Martin glanced at Annette, and, distracted by her fiery energy, fast pace, and delicate beauty, realized that this day was important to her. At once, he realized that he was being given something, even though he had no idea exactly what.

Alistair, alighting from a carriage, grinned at Martin. Elizabeth, happy to be somewhere she could contribute something besides a menu, walked with Annette toward the station building.

The milk station was one block north of the Waltham Watch Factory, the city's main employer, located on 74 Rumford Street. The single one-story wooden building had been constructed through funds raised by Elizabeth and Alfred, Annette recalled, in order to provide milk and prepared food for babies. Since the building could only accommodate a handful of people, a line of women carrying infants and accompanied by young children had gathered outside the station. Already at work distributing eight-and-one-half-quart cans of fresh cows' milk from local farmers to mothers, Charlotte Macleod and a senior pupil nurse from the Waltham Training School for Nurses were engaged in their well-executed distribution routine.

Charlotte taught mothers how to pour milk from the can, tilting it carefully, using the handle on one side. She then lifted the turned wooden stopple, stressing the need to meticulously clean the stopple, since its porous structure might harbor germs, therefore contaminating the milk and harming the baby. After Charlotte's instruction, the pupil nurse discussed how to feed the baby, when to begin food supplements such as pap—breadcrumbs cooked in milk—or panada—bread cooked in broth—and the importance of overall cleanliness.

Knowing that he was wildly out of his element, Martin cleared his throat and asked if mothers still employed wet nurses.

Annette replied first. "Wet nursing remains an option for mothers unable to breastfeed, or for women whose husbands forbid the practice. However, worries that wet nurses may encourage use of Godfrey's Cordial, an opiate called *Quietness*, to soothe colicky babies has dramatically reduced the use of these important women."

Elizabeth added that many women were now employed in cities, working in businesses such as the Watch Factory. She gestured to the building across the street.

"Working women," she said, "could, on average, purchase an eight-and-one-half-quart can of cow's milk for twenty-four cents." For women unable to pay for the milk, Elizabeth indicated that they received the milk at no cost. The Waltham milk station was established as a local charity, dealing with local farmers rather than those in the Milk Producers' Union, an association serving to self-regulate business practices for legal, ethical, and safety standards. As a charity, the local farmers set their own rules according to community needs.

"Martin," said Annette, "the milk station serves as an outpatient health education center associated with Waltham Hospital." Expanding, she noted that Charlotte, pupil nurses, Elizabeth, and she had been trained by Alfred to assess for common problems such as malnutrition, vitamin deficiencies, failure to thrive, and other minor illnesses. Mothers, she added, would sometimes ask for advice on childcare, immunizations, how to lift depression, prevention of pregnancy, or managing unruly husbands.

"Our milk station distributes milk," continued Elizabeth, "but it is also an education and referral center, sometimes encouraging mothers to bring their children to a pediatrician, a new type of doctor specializing in childcare." Elizabeth linked decreasing infant and child morbidity and mortality to efforts such as milk stations and immunizations. She looked intently at Martin as she concluded. "Health education of the public is the key to our nation's health."

The small crowd at the milk station suddenly began clamoring for help, as two women lifted another off the ground, placing her against the outside wall of the building. Eyes closed, with shallow and rapid breathing, the young woman had fainted, dropping her infant to the ground. The infant cried, signaling a live child — a welcome sound to Charlotte, who had rushed outside to help.

"Her pulse is rapid, and she feels very warm. Let's get her inside in the shade. Once she comes to, we can give her water." Charlotte gestured for Martin, who had sprinted quickly to her side, to gather up the infant and follow her. Inside, Charlotte and the pupil nurse placed the woman on the cool concrete floor, lifting her head onto a towel-wrapped milk can. Once awake, the young woman eagerly drank the water, thanking the group for their help. At seventeen years of age, the mother admitted that she had little food and was unable to breastfeed her two-month-old infant. "The baby," she said, "cannot latch on."

Charlotte arranged for the young mother's infant to be evaluated at Waltham Hospital, with possible treatment in the baby unit. Once the mother and infant had recovered, Elizabeth thanked Martin for his assistance, adding that situations such as this occurred frequently enough to warrant establishment of a hospital for babies, or, perhaps more useful, a hospital specializing in childcare under management by pediatricians. "Such a hospital," Charlotte added, "is a place that Alfred wants these mothers to have."

By noon, the group concluded their tour of the milk station and, after a light lunch prepared by Elizabeth, planned to visit sick babies at Waltham Hospital.

Martin's curiosity, however, had been piqued by Elizabeth's comments about women working in city factories.

"May we consider visiting the watch factory across the street? Do they have a need for care at this factory? I wonder if they have work injuries that require immediate attention." Annette, pleased at Martin's interest, asked the group if a detour to the factory was acceptable. Although she needed to remain at the milk station, Charlotte brightened at Martin's suggestion.

"At our school, we have just begun a course in industrial nursing," she reported, "with pupils sent for a month to learn under the leadership of one of our graduates, Bessie Frawley, working at the watch factory. We plan to expand to another site, the Hood Rubber Company in Watertown, under the supervision of Eugenia French, another one of our graduates. You will find these factories to be excellent sites for pupil instruction. They learn practical skills in injury management as well as what we call three-second critical thinking, or emergency management." She urged Martin to ask to meet with Bessie Frawley at the front door, seeking a tour of the factory along with a description of health services rendered at her office.

Surprised and delighted by Martin's desire to visit the watch factory, Annette and her colleagues decided to reschedule a visit to the baby unit for another day.

Bessie, thrilled to tour Martin, Annette, Elizabeth, and Alistair through the watch factory, provided an overview of the company, describing the watchmaking crafts undertaken by several hundred employees on site. Given occasional work injuries, as well as common illnesses, Bessie said that she was busy every day with wound care, health education, or illness checks. Seeing an opportunity with this visit, Bessie added that the clinic could provide additional health promotion services if a second nurse were recruited.

Annette, Alistair, and Elizabeth, elated by their eventful day, thanked Martin for joining them, and encouraged him to visit the Waltham Hospital and Training School when his calendar would allow it.

"It was my pleasure to join you today. The scales continue to fall from my eyes." Martin smiled at his new colleagues, shaking hands with all three.

"I am certainly beginning to understand your point now about nurse education. There is more here than simply following doctors' orders in hospitals. I need to learn more about how existing and planned legislation aligns with all I saw today. I'll begin by studying our State Board of Health, its mission and goals. Then, I'll review medicine's registration board and any bills that have been proposed for nursing." Before turning away, he asked for a private moment with Annette.

"Annette, it will soon be July 4th, Independence Day. Would you care to join me," he continued, flashing a wicked grin, "in celebrating our country's independence from British tyranny?"

"Absolutely!" Smiling broadly and shaking Martin's hand again, Annette saw Alistair grinning in the background.

"Good, I'll pick you up at noon at your home!" Jumping into the carriage, Martin said goodbye with a jaunty wave.

"Well, my friend, you have snagged a winner," Alistair whispered as he helped Annette into their carriage. He could not contain his happiness for his dear friend.

Charles, grateful that the July 4th holiday would fall on a Saturday and thus would not interrupt business, was not looking forward to his late afternoon meeting with the deans of the medical and dental schools. He conceded that his wife, Grace, had been correct at breakfast. He was both grumpy and edgy.

On the subject of a Harvard school of nursing, he knew that he could not predict his new dental school dean's reactions.

Today he would introduce the plan to establish a school of nursing in the near future. He wondered if his three-legged stool metaphor would aptly characterize the interrelationships among medicine, dentistry, and nursing in modern-day health care. While he easily predicted the endorsement of William Richardson, dean of the medical school, Charles was not convinced that Eugene Smith, dean of the dental school, would approve of university resources possibly spilling over to educate nurses. Did not all women nurse by nature? Following such lines of logic, perhaps Smith would be content with a two-legged stool.

Smith was appointed dean upon the death of his predecessor, Thomas H. Chandler, a Harvard-trained lawyer and graduate of Harvard College, who had served twenty-one years as dean. Both educational pragmatists espousing science and technology, Charles and Chandler read the political tea leaves quickly, averting disasters before others realized the steamroller was ready to crush them. Oh, how I miss Chandler, Charles thought. Smith, on the other hand, was an expert dental clinician, the single most skilled person he sought when he had a toothache. But Smith's world was a small one, whereas Chandler's had been expansive. Would Smith, a venal man, consider a nursing school an arrogant upstart, forcing his young school into a less favored position alongside women?

Considering tactics, Charles saw Smith's truculence as an opening to the conversation.

Richardson, a tall, thin, meticulously groomed middle-aged man with short, cropped hair and a receding hairline, vigorously shook Charles's hand. He was a long-term colleague of Charles, curious about the reason for a meeting on the eve of Boston's most cherished secular holiday. Whatever the reason, Richardson trusted Charles's leadership, and more importantly, his instincts for change.

In contrast, Smith was a shorter, more rotund man, with bushy eyebrows, thick graying hair and a painter's brush mustache. Frequently angling his round eyeglass frame on his nose, Smith was uncomfortable, fidgety in his chair. He, too, was quite interested in this meeting with Harvard's president. Knowing that he did not have the gravitas of either Eliot or Richardson, Smith, appointed as dean only one year earlier, was aware that he served at the pleasure of the president.

Both deans waited for Charles to speak.

"We have one goal left at Harvard regarding health. We must prepare students in nursing to work with you," Charles waved his arm toward Richardson and Smith, "to keep our citizens healthy. Together with nursing, your professions are the proverbial three-legged stool."

Richardson smiled in agreement with Charles. "Absolutely correct!" he added. "There is enough illness in our population to welcome nurses to our team. I say that Harvard should be the first to award nurses a university degree." Charles smiled broadly, recalling that a few years ago he had told Alfred that Richardson, ever a progressive, was always quick to get on board the bandwagon.

"Eugene, what are your thoughts?" asked Charles, eyebrows slightly cocked.

"Yes, of course," Smith said, "when will such a new school begin?"

"The approval process, both formal and informal, starts with you. I need my medical and dental deans to support a new partner. Support from faculty, alumni, legislators, hospital administrators, industry leaders, and others will be sought over time." Charles then expanded on the background to his goal, describing the recently approved degree-granting authority to Radcliffe College and the professionalization of nursing that had been ongoing for the past two decades.

Charles concluded his background summary with what he knew to be his ace up his sleeve, the 1883 Harvard Medical School alumnus, Alfred Worcester.

"Alfred," exclaimed Richardson, "I haven't seen him in years!"

Richardson, Assistant Professor of Obstetrics at Harvard when Alfred was a medical student, had placed Alfred in charge of both patient care and the nursing staff at the Boston Lying-In Hospital.

"Alfred's work at the Lying-In was beyond comparison. In fact, he started a nursing school there shortly after organizing medical record documentation and establishing sanitary conditions. He is a good doctor, and perhaps an even better teacher. When he finished his rotation at the Lying-In, the nursing staff honored him with a grand party. They even gave him an umbrella with his name carved on an ivory handle. Alfred is a serious man."

Unlike Richardson, Smith did not know Alfred, and it would not have mattered if he had. Smith had only financial concerns.

"Charles, how will the nursing school be financed?" Smith, continuously seeking funds for expansion of his school, particularly since it's expansion to a three-year curriculum in 1891, worried that the new school might be established at the expense of his budget.

"Well, Eugene, we have the usual array of revenue sources, including tuition and fees, gifts, and endowments. At present, I am courting two potential endowment donors, well in advance of the school's start."

Charles walked slowly to the large window overlooking the Harvard Yard.

"I need you to publicly support the new School of Nursing." Turning to them, he asked, "Will you do that?"

Richardson assured Charles that he, his faculty, and the medical school alumni would graciously support the nursing school.

"And dentistry, Eugene?" questioned Charles.

"You have my support, but with a condition," said Smith. "I need concrete evidence that you will continue to support my school to the level that is needed for excellence. My school is not yet thirty years old, and we need five additional faculty lines in specialty fields, in addition to more space, in the next two years. Will you consider this request?" Smith, surprised by his own language, sat and began fidgeting with his pen.

Ever the negotiator, Charles bargained downward. "Would three new faculty lines and appropriate office and laboratory space for them be an adequate offer to secure your support?"

Smith agreed that Charles's offer would garner his and his faculty's support. However, he could not promise support from alumni, many of whom had worked under Nathan Cooley Keep, the first dean appointed in 1867. "The Keep Alumni," as Smith called them, "feel that the school and university have abandoned their original objectives, supporting programs not as relevant as dentistry."

Charles assured Smith that there was time to galvanize the dental alumni and to appropriately thank them for their loyalty to Harvard and to the nation's dental health. Perhaps a gala in the near future, Charles thought, held to honor the alumni of the dental and medical schools.

"Look," said Charles, gesturing to the window and, beyond it, Harvard Yard, "they are putting up tents and lawn chairs for the holiday event tomorrow. Will you both be attending? All of our schools' alumni have been invited to a generous cookout, with the university band and fireworks scheduled to celebrate at sunset, and music all day. Do you like watermelon?" Pointing to a large two-horse-drawn wagon loaded with watermelons, Charles gestured to his guests to watch as the melons were unloaded onto tables for the next day.

"Enjoy this lovely holiday, gentlemen!" Relieved, Charles returned home to Grace, less grumpy than when he had left.

It was already eighty-eight degrees by mid-morning on July 4th, and Martin found the two horses pulling his hansom carriage distracted by the steam arising from the streets. His thoughts had turned to Annette.

Annette had graduated from Radcliffe College with her Master of Arts in ancient languages only two weeks ago. While he had not been invited to her graduation, he realized the intellectual prowess of this woman who had plowed through an AB degree in 1894 and moved directly to an AM in 1896. And now, it seemed, she was moving on to something entirely different. She was quite unlike any other woman he had known or would likely ever know.

Trading his stiff lawyer suit for looser attire, Martin had selected a deep-gray belted, single-breasted tweed Norfolk jacket with box pleats on front and back. His breeches, lying slightly below his knees, met long, black knee-high stockings and low-heeled black Oxonian shoes. Appropriately attired for an afternoon with an educated Back Bay woman, Martin looked forward to his planned picnic with Annette at Harvard Yard, a distance of approximately a half mile from her home on Massachusetts Avenue. Given congestion on this holiday, Martin's alternate plan was to simply spread his picnic blanket on a shaded patch under the Washington Elm tree in Cambridge Common, even closer to her home.

Glancing quickly at the picnic basket on the carriage floor, Martin felt proud of his choices. Considering Annette's passion for good health, Martin had packed apples, bananas, sandwiches of grated cheese with nuts and lettuce, and glazed blueberry scones for dessert. With a bottle of sweet Riesling wine and two crystal wine flutes packed securely, Martin was hopeful that this picnic would be remembered.

Caroline opened the door upon Martin's arrival. Ever elegant and gracious, she waved him into their foyer, asking that he take a seat in the parlor while she announced his arrival to Annette.

"What a pleasure to meet you, Martin! Annette has spoken highly of you over the past few weeks. She is very pleased that you are so interested in nursing and health care," said Caroline as she placed his boater straw hat and riding gloves on a receiving table in the foyer. "Before she comes downstairs, I want to invite you to bring her home right after the fireworks at sunset. She made me promise to not have a big party celebrating her second Radcliffe graduation, but I do want to surprise her with a small late evening dessert party when you come home. Is that acceptable to you, Martin?"

"Absolutely wonderful!" Martin exclaimed, grateful to have been invited to the celebration so early in their dating relationship. While his planned late sunset walk around the park would have to be rescheduled, the opportunity to meet Annette's family and intimate friends would be an unexpected delight.

In her bedroom, Annette sat patiently in her desk chair as Marguerite swept her long hair into a classic Gibson Girl silhouette, creating a relatively messy, yet contained, updo framing her delicate face, with flimsy tendrils dropping from her temples. Wearing white bloomers, a light-blue flouncy blouse, a large red-ribbon necktie, and black Edwardian laced leather shoes, Annette felt patriotic. Sporting a crimson ribbon threaded through her hairdo, she was also proud of both her alma mater, Radcliffe, and its parent institution, Harvard. Remembering her Aunt Ellen, Annette stashed a pack of Vanity Fair cigarettes and a box of Diamond matches into a large, hidden pocket in her bloomers.

Determined to enjoy Martin's company without thoughts of tomorrow, Annette smiled, eagerly taking his hand to embark in the carriage. Annette wondered what she was not privy to as she caught Martin's wink at Caroline as they drove away.

Wink or no wink, let this marvelous day link my education to my future, thought Annette as she settled next to Martin, smelling the delicious aromas from his picnic basket. For her contribution, Annette carried a large, thick red blanket to spread on the grass, the color making them noticeable from any angle in Harvard Yard.

"Martin, you cannot imagine how happy I am today."

"As am I," said Martin, smiling as they arrived at Harvard Yard. Helping Annette from the carriage and then lifting out the picnic basket, Martin spread her red blanket on a patch of thick grass under the shade of an oak tree. With the band playing "America the Beautiful," lyrics from the 1893 poem by Katharine Lee Bates, Annette and Martin laid on the blanket, looking at the blue sky, loosely holding hands. Martin, generally a chatterbox, fell silent. Annette quietly hummed the patriotic song, reminding her of the Chicago World's Fair, a pivotal event in her life.

Acting Governor Roger Wolcott was escorted to the stage's podium as Bates completed her reading, the band respectfully silent behind him. Wolcott, governor since March, upon the death of Frederic T. Greenhalge, sporting wavy white hair combed straight back with accompanying walrus-style beard, was a Harvard Law School graduate with appointments as trustee of the Massachusetts General Hospital and the Eye and Ear Infirmary. As revelers were urged to silence, Wolcott slowly recited the Declaration of Independence in his strong tenor voice. As he recited, volunteers at makeshift stands draped with American flags, preparing cold drinks made from camellia, Darjeeling, and Earl Grey teas, stopped to listen.

"No Independence Day celebration is complete without a tea party," exclaimed one volunteer, handing Annette and Martin cold tea drinks at the completion of Wolcott's recitation. Now 8:30 pm, they returned to their picnic blanket to watch the fireworks, the grand finale.

The fireworks began slowly, with Roman candles soaring first in white, then in red and blue. Then the pinwheels began, a spectacular swirl of American flag colors lighting up the sky. The sound and smoke increased, the crackles and whistles turning to loud bangs. And then it seemed as if the sky exploded in a final salute sounding like artillery shells exploding, with light flooding Cambridge Commons. Martin looked at Annette looking at the sky and held his breath as his heart leaped toward her.

Annette, wanting to prolong the evening, was surprised when Martin said that he had promised to return her home shortly after the fireworks. Crestfallen, she hoped they might have another charming day together before she began nursing school. She wondered if he would be a memory or a presence.

Annette's home on Massachusetts Avenue was dark, with window shades drawn, no light escaping around drape edges. Surprised, Annette alighted from the carriage with Martin, placing the picnic blanket on a porch swing. Martin knocked on one of the two panels to the Mahogany front door, anticipating loud cheering as they entered.

The door was open. They entered noiselessly.

Becoming slightly concerned, Annette called for her mother and father, wondering if they might still be in town celebrating with friends.

As she crossed over to the main sitting parlor, the room exploded with light, cheering, chatter, piano music, singing, all immersed in the delicious aroma of gardenias.

Caroline and Amos hugged Annette, congratulating her for graduating from Radcliffe College with her Master of Arts degree with honors. In the background, Marguerite and Elizabeth Worcester provided a musical interlude with piano and singing, and Elizabeth Agassiz and Charles Eliot poured champagne into Waterford Lismore toasting flute glasses, as Stubby held them securely. Alfred and Charlotte arranged a few gift packages on a side bar table, placing them in some apparent order of relevance while Millie and Alistair remained at the entrance, ceremoniously holding the two doors open as Martin gave his picnic basket to the kitchen staff. Matthew Campbell, Alistair's father, lingered at an appetizer table, taste-testing finger tea sandwiches, deviled quail eggs, various cheese bites, corn bread sticks, relishes, and cooked shrimp.

Surprised, tired, embarrassed, and elated, Annette held Martin's hand tightly, unsure of next steps. Never one for attention, she thanked everyone for sharing this wonderful day with her and, turning to her mother, kissed her warmly, thanking her for this very unexpected party.

"We are all very proud of you, dear Annie. Please enjoy your success." Caroline, moving closer to Annette, whispered, "Thank you, my dear daughter, for changing my life as well."

Elizabeth Agassiz passed out champagne glasses as Charles toasted Annette, announcing that she was the first woman integral to planning a Harvard school, and might, once she completed her nursing program, make a Harvard school of nursing a reality in the twentieth century.

Walled in by Charles, Elizabeth, Alfred, and friends, Annette suddenly felt overwhelmed by the enormity of nursing and her future in it. They have more faith in me than I have, she thought, worried equally of success and of failure. If we succeed, then success must follow success. If we fail, then I have failed. While success will be shared, failure will be mine.

As such thoughts washed over her, she stiffened, imperceptibly so. Martin reached for her hand. While he knew that he might never really know this woman, he was getting a sense of her, of the little ways she responded to those around her.

"Charles is only recalling what you have done and will do," he whispered as he turned his lips near her ear. Martin's confidence bolstered Annette. He was thrilling.

Pointing to the gift table, Martin handed Annette one of the gifts wrapped so lovingly for her. She opened Alfred and Charlotte's gift first, eyes sparkling at the gold wrapping paper and bright crimson flower adorning it.

"You will use this the rest of your life, Annette," said Charlotte, excitedly. Anxious to give Annette a meaningful gift, Charlotte and Alfred had selected a sterling silver nurse watch fob with chain attachment to loop on either a collar or a waist belt. "A necessity for nurses," said Charlotte proudly, wrapping her arm around Annette. Alfred, holding the fob watch, asked if Annette needed a demonstration on how to attach it to clothing. For a moment, Annette caught her breath, feeling how close Alfred was to her.

Fastening the watch in one quick movement, Alfred moved back from her and next to Charlotte. Again, Martin reached for her hand.

Opening the next gift, Annette felt relief, almost peacefulness. I can let Alfred go now, she thought. I must and I will. She beamed at each present, especially the little white sandals Millie had given her. "The Winged Sandals of Hermes," Millie had written on the card.

"Am I now to deliver messages between humans and the divine?" Annette asked.

"As you have been doing all along," Millie replied as she hugged her friend.

In early September, Annette would enter the Waltham Training School, with graduation in late spring, 1898. Here she was, beginning again.

Stubby, raising his champagne glass, asked if a second toast could be tolerated.

Hearing assent, Stubby asked his sister Caroline to refill guests' glasses as he fiddled with his eyeglasses, pulling a small piece of paper from his pants pocket.

"My beloved Ellen died this year, and as you may recall from past holiday celebrations, Ellen would conclude July fourth parties with a toast to her grandfather, Theodore Sedgwick, who fought as a United States general during the American Revolution and served in both the Massachusetts Senate and House of Representatives for many years. She saluted his courage, his dedication to country and family, and his unflinching passion to end slavery. Like her grandfather, Ellen championed freedom. Women's right to vote, their right to education and careers, their right to contribute to society, and yes, even their right to smoke."

Enjoying the chuckles in the room, Stubby concluded, tears in his eyes.

"We must vow to finish Ellen's work."

"To Ellen!" Stubby toasted his wife, with all in the room cheering.

As guests prepared to leave, Annette walked Martin into the backyard, to the safe place where Ellen first introduced her to the world in which she now lived. As she lit a Vanity Fair cigarette, passing it to Martin, Annette asked if it was possible that she would see him as she shuffled back and forth to Waltham.

"More than possible, my dear Annette, it is very probable." She thought of her aunt and took his hand in hers. They sat in silence until the last guest had left.

Origin

"Arthur," said Alfred, "both the Waltham Hospital and Training School are growing quickly. Our services are expanding too quickly for our present buildings."

Comfortable in the nurses' parlor of the training school, sipping tea and sitting between Charlotte and his friend Arthur Lyman, Alfred updated Arthur on space needs of both the hospital and school. Twenty-three years the physician's senior, Arthur was a very successful cotton manufacturer, holding both AB and AM degrees from Harvard University. A quiet, reticent businessman, Arthur served as an overseer at his alma mater, a role integral to planned growth of the institution.

Arthur understood space well. He resided yearlong at the Lyman Estate in Waltham, among carefully landscaped gardens and shaded porches. Often called *The Vale* by local residents due to its location between a wooded rocky ridge and a brook, the building was constructed in 1798 by Arthur's grandfather, Theodore Lyman, a slave trader in the West Indies who began exporting furs to China when the Supreme Judicial Court of Massachusetts ruled in 1783 that slavery was unconstitutional in the commonwealth.

Occasionally, *The Vale* hosted conferences and community meetings, as well as educators, lawyers, and politicians.

Downplaying his wealth and its origin, Arthur's appearance was plain, his philanthropy generous. Average height with thinning gray hair and clean-shaven, he typically wore straight black trousers, a short waistcoat and a white shirt with a stiff collar and black bowtie. Alfred first met Arthur at a conference for doctors and hospital administrators held at *The Vale* several years earlier. Fascinated with advances in science and health, Arthur quickly bonded with Alfred, captivated both by his drive to cure tuberculosis and his passion for improved obstetrical care.

At Alfred's invitation, Arthur had toured both the hospital and the nursing school, still housed in the home of Edward Cutler. Deeply impressed with the care delivered to patients by the doctors and pupil nurses, Arthur now pledged his commitment to help fund a new, expanded training school and nurses' home, one to accommodate anticipated growth needs. Alfred and Charlotte were heartened at his generosity. Arthur waved thanks away and changed the subject.

Catching him off guard, Arthur asked Alfred, "Do you know what Charlie is planning regarding nurses' training at Harvard?"

Arthur seemed eager to discuss nursing. He explained that Charles had recently made a presentation at an overseers meeting about a possible new school, a Harvard school of nursing. Alfred and Charlotte were silenced by Arthur's extensive knowledge of work they had sponsored.

"I don't have many details, but I appreciate the wonderful enthusiasm." Expanding, Arthur indicated that Charles had spoken of the need for medicine, dentistry, and nursing. Arthur reported Charles's saying that, without educated nurses, the three-legged health stool is incomplete. "He seems fixed," Arthur said with a grin, "on that image."

"Alfred, I am sure that you have heard of my cousin's plans, am I correct? How will Charlie's plan impact the Waltham Training School for Nurses? Will you still want to construct a new nursing building if Harvard establishes a school of nursing?" An efficient businessman, Arthur was direct.

"Your *cousin*?" Alfred was bewildered.

Alfred felt foolish that he had not known that Arthur and Charles were first cousins, that Charles's mother and Arthur's father were siblings, and uninformed that his friend knew so much about plans for nursing at Harvard. Pivot quickly, he thought. With so many connections to draw upon, Alfred now swiveled to a new plan.

After apologizing for his slowness in connecting Charles and Arthur as cousins, Alfred described their ongoing work for a school of nursing and agreed that the plan for Harvard was intimately associated with the Waltham School. Over the next hour, Alfred described those who were making Charles's ideas a reality, ending with the target date of 1900 for founding of the Harvard School.

"The Waltham School will transition to the Harvard School in 1900, just as the baccalaureate program begins and the last class is admitted to Waltham. This timing would allow the last Waltham class to graduate in 1903 and the first Harvard students to graduate in 1904. There would be no interruption in graduation of nurses for our communities." Alfred also discussed the curriculum, clinical rotations, the change from apprenticeship training to education, and finances associated with college education. He decided to be as direct as would his friend.

"Arthur, would you consider supporting a Harvard school of nursing to help us transition to collegiate education for nurses at our own alma mater?" Alfred was more straightforward than Arthur believed possible, and Charlotte tensed at the question.

"Alfred, let me tell you something about the grandfather Charles and I share. In addition to including Charles in his will, my grandfather gave him a special legacy gift, a financial provision in his will to offset any misfortune he might have faced as an adult due to the large birthmark on the right side of his face." Alfred had, until that moment, never considered Charles as burdened by anything on earth but then realized that, in 1834, the family only saw an infant facing a world that hated deformity.

"So, you see," Arthur continued, "my grandfather, much like me, loved Charlie. Thought he was special. He would have loved to live long enough to see what he has accomplished at Harvard." Arthur did not say that his grandfather also left a legacy of cruelty that would haunt both grandchildren throughout their lives.

Taking a breath, Arthur, ever concrete, asked, "Well, what amount of financial support are you seeking?"

Alfred answered the amount of funding sought would depend on the number of committed financial supporters. Arthur repeated that Charles informed the overseers that he hoped to build a nursing school on the Longwood Campus, to be adjacent with the medical school. Buildings, Arthur knew, took money.

"Alfred, who is Charlie lining up to ask for endowments?"

Standing up from his armchair in the school's parlor, Alfred began pacing, unsure if it was appropriate to discuss Charles's funding plans with his own benefactor. Charlotte had come to know this behavior all too well and left the room, giving Alfred the privacy he needed.

Alfred decided to reveal two other possible sources of funding once Charlotte had left the room. One possible donor, Matthew Campbell, was a devoted Harvard overseer, as was Arthur, and eager to broaden the scope and impact of Harvard nationally. Years earlier, Matthew had voiced his interest in naming a professorship in the arts, an endowment that might now shift to either support of Radcliffe College or to a future school of nursing. Alfred added that he hoped Matthew would support the nursing school, with an endowment for Radcliffe College to be sought from Alice Mary Longfellow.

"There is another possible donor, but quite unlike others." Alfred briefly described the banker and philanthropist Jacob Schiff. From his recollection of descriptions provided by Annette and Millie, Alfred added that Schiff believed in *Tzedakah,* a view of charity as a path to the achievement of social justice.

"Charles, Annette, Charlotte, and I will visit Jacob Schiff late this summer. Charles plans on suggesting his support for an endowed professorship in public health nursing, given his passion for family and community health."

"Alfred, you and Charlie can count on me. I will transfer my pledge of financial support for the Waltham School to the Harvard School, once it is approved by the state legislature."

Shaking hands with Alfred, Arthur asked that he be kept updated on progress on the Harvard School.

"I will keep my ears to the ground. I'll let you know if I think of other possible donors." Predictably understated, Arthur flashed an endearing smile at his junior colleague, tipping his hat ever so slightly, as he left the parlor.

Charles and Alfred walked up the three steps to the impressive glass-paneled mahogany double doors of Harvard House, a three-story crimson-red brick and Indiana limestone building opened only two years earlier at 27 West Forty-Fourth Street, nestled between Fifth and Sixth Avenues in midtown New York City.

It was Friday, October 23, 1896 — a chilly day with a boundless blue sky. Charles removed his gloves and smiled at Alfred as he held open the front door, ushering him into one of the two small adjoining reception rooms, opening to a grill room in the rear that overlooked a garden. Tastefully decorated with small pumpkins and fall foliage adorning the fireplace mantles, the interior was furnished entirely with donations from members. The posh club had been founded in 1865 by graduates wishing to continue the fellowship they had experienced in Cambridge. Despite Charles's passion for Harvard's usefulness and practicality, Harvard House symbolized aristocracy and elitism, rather than merit.

As they entered, an older man in formal gentleman's daywear, wearing a ditto suit of matching black jacket, trousers, and waistcoat, approached them, handing each a Cuban cigar from Ybor City, Florida, that had an irresistible sweet smell of tobacco and cedar.

"One of our alumni asked that I distribute these to all that enter the House. He purchased them while on a trip to Florida." After pointing them to the staircase that would bring them to the library, the doorman retired to a reception room.

Charles seems uncomfortable, almost out of place here, Alfred thought.

"We will meet Jacob Schiff in this library. It is quite spacious. Since the House does not have a kitchen, I have ordered a light lunch to be delivered for our meeting." As Alfred sat on one of the large velvet-upholstered couches, Charles scanned the room, noting several comfortable chairs but a dearth of library holdings. Frowning to himself, Charles adjusted his round, wire-rimmed eyeglasses and explored the books lining two bookshelves, one on either side of the fireplace. Surely, he hoped, their holdings would expand in time. For now, the spacious, secluded room was lovely for casual reading of newspapers and popular journals. A haven for Harvard graduates living or working in New York City with time to spare for light reading and even lighter conversation. Charles equally hoped that the room would not become a place for privileged Harvard graduates to lounge while knowing nothing of the responsibility that comes with privilege.

Alfred, eager to meet Jacob, had been primed by Annette and Millie of his support of Lillian Wald, her Henry Street Settlement, and accompanying visiting nurse services. Grateful that Charles's request to meet Lillian and tour the neighborhood served by her visiting nurses had been received positively, Alfred looked forward to sharing information with Jacob about the Waltham Training School's similar rotations in the community. As Charles knew, Alfred shared Jacob's concerns about community health.

While Charles knew that Matthew Campbell was very likely to endow a dedicated building for the Harvard School of Nursing, other funding would also be needed. In particular, funding for influential professorships, such as Francis J. Child's Boylston Professor of Rhetoric and Oratory, would also be needed. Gazing at Alfred again, Charles thought of their visit the next day to Lillian Wald, Schiff's champion of public health in the Lower East Side.

Perhaps, he wondered, an endowed professorship in public health nursing might be the best direction.

Charles recalled to Alfred Jacob's 1890 gift for the establishment of a Harvard Semitic Museum. With construction targeted for completion in 1903, the Semitic holdings were temporarily housed in a gallery of the new addition to the Peabody Museum on Divinity Avenue on the Harvard campus. He wanted Alfred to understand that Jacob was generous but that his gifts always had a purpose, such as the study of ancient cultures and histories of people who spoke Semitic languages.

"Alfred, our approach with Jacob must be the value of nurses to the public's health. He is supporting Lillian Wald's initiatives that improve the lives of the Jewish community in the Lower East Side. We cannot forget that." Continuing, Charles urged Alfred to avoid talk of hospitals and surgical advancements, to focus instead on health education, immunization efforts, obstetrical improvements, and family care.

"Jacob's passion is people, not hospitals. If Jacob believed that more hospitals would help people, then he would have already funded more."

Alfred relaxed almost immediately upon meeting Jacob. Wearing a charcoal-colored frock coat falling to his knees, along with a five-button vest straining to retain his girth and a starched white shirt with black tie, Jacob was an affable, genial businessman at ease in Harvard House if for no other reason than that he knew that banking secured a chair for him in any room. Sitting in an armchair opposite Charles, Jacob occasionally smoothed his white Verdi-style beard and mustache away from his Cuban cigar, stating that the cigar alone was worth his trip from the financial district in Lower Manhattan to Midtown.

"Generally, Charles, the Cambridge set invites me to dine with them when they want — or need — something." Always one step ahead, he knew the backgrounds and intentions of those with whom he met. Eyes twinkling, Jacob sipped his deep-dish vegetable soup, crunching an occasional oyster cracker. Because Lillian said he must watch his weight, he had declined a sandwich or stew.

Understanding exactly the conversation that Jacob was framing, Charles did not waste time getting to the reason for their visit.

"Science is advancing quickly. Medicine is following suit." Charles noted that a cascade was developing in the country. First, hospital construction. Second, establishment of training schools of nursing operated by hospitals. And lastly, a subtle shift in focus from health care of people and communities to illness care delivered in hospitals.

"This shift," he continued, "has a dangerous, unanticipated outcome. Pupil nurses are not educated. They experience only apprenticeship in a system that hinders learning. Hospitals, doctors, administrators get rich at the expense of pupil nurses, held hostage to hospital monopoly."

Charles concluded, "Nurses play an important role in health care, particularly in community and public health. They need college education, as do physicians and dentists."

"Harvard must establish a school of nursing." The final point now acknowledged, Charles asked Jacob if he might consider financially supporting some part of Harvard's new school.

"Before I respond, Charles, I would like to hear from Alfred. You are a doctor operating a training school. Do you offer your program as Charles describes? In the hospital model? Or do you educate your pupils differently?"

Alfred, on cue though taken aback at Jacob's knowledge of his work, provided a short description of the Waltham Hospital and Training School for Nurses, stressing the program's emphasis on health promotion in many settings, including hospitals, homes, industry, outpatient clinics, or any place where people live and work.

"We hope to transition our training school over to the Harvard School of Nursing. Once the college program begins, we will enter our last class and close the school once these students graduate." Alfred concluded, saying that he looked forward to meeting Lillian Wald the next day, hoping to learn more about her visiting nurse services in the Lower East Side.

"Give me a day to consider your request. I agree with what you have said, and I agree with a Harvard school of nursing. I'll be at the Henry Street Settlement in the morning. I will share my thoughts about your request at that time." With a sure handshake, Jacob bid farewell to Charles and Alfred, stepped into his hansom cab, and returned to Kuhn, Loeb and Company.

As they returned to their rooms at the elegant Brunswick Hotel, located at the juncture between Madison Square Park and Fifth Avenue between Twenty-Sixth and Twenty-Seventh Streets in Midtown, Charles and Alfred were cautiously optimistic that Jacob Schiff would agree to financially support some aspect of a new Harvard school of nursing. Securing Lillian Wald's favor, Charles knew, would be critical. Grateful that Annette and Charlotte would be joining them tomorrow, Charles and Alfred considered an endowed professorship of public health nursing as the most viable gift to seek from Jacob.

Annette, Charles mused, is our trump card.

In the three years since Annette first met Lillian Wald, much had changed. Lillian and her friend, Mary Brewster, had relocated from their tenement building on Jefferson Street into 265 Henry Street in summer, 1895. The building, purchased for their use by Jacob Schiff, had been recently enlarged with a full third floor to accommodate nine nurses in addition to Lillian and Mary. Mrs. McRae and her son, Tommie, had moved in with Lillian and Mary, loyal to the women and deeply dedicated to their work. Schiff also provided funding for refurbishments to the property, giving Lillian freedom to outfit the building as she deemed appropriate.

Annette had also changed.

Once accepted to the Waltham Training School for Nurses in fall 1896, Annette became a Brownie, wearing the mandatory brown and white checked gingham uniform, in the program's new, six-month preparatory course. Dressing on the very first day, she took pride as she looped onto her belt the nurse watch fob that Alfred and Charlotte had given her. Once the course was completed in winter 1897, she would don her regular pupil uniform, a blue and white striped gingham with a bib apron and surplice supplies waist pocket, a reminder of the ideals of the profession, according to school staff. Since pupils were given the materials for Brownie uniforms, her mother Caroline arranged for the family seamstress to sew hers, a privilege Annette kept secret from the other students, in addition to her degrees from Radcliffe College.

During their train ride from Boston to New York City, Annette delicately discussed the Waltham School preparation course with Charlotte, cautious not to offend her, critically aware of the differences in the lived experiences between them. Reviewing her notes in the journal that Amos had given her at the family's late summer party in celebration of her enrollment in Waltham's nursing program, Annette silently giggled at her own comment that the new Harvard curriculum should discontinue the preparatory course.

Charlotte can never see this comment, Annette thought.

Sanitary science and principles of cleanliness, along with nutritious cooking and sewing, had been traditionally embraced as nursing practice by nurse leaders.

Cooking and cleaning, however, were not nursing duties to Annette. Rather, Annette wrote in her journal, such are responsibilities of all people. Or, if resources were available, job responsibilities of employees, possibly kitchen maids, housekeepers, lady's maids, butlers, footmen, or valets. Surely, she had written, all responsible adults can manage their own cleanliness and food needs.

Charlotte, however, assured Annette that nursing superintendents who were members of the American Society for Superintendents for Training Schools of Nursing strongly advocated for closely supervised preparatory courses, given that not all entering pupils sufficiently understood the values of cleanliness in the home. Hesitantly, Charlotte described most pupil nurses as women from different classes than Annette. Framing Annette as unique, both in her education and the privileges of her homelife, Charlotte urged her to be patient.

"Your curriculum, Annette, will not include the duties you are now doing as a Brownie. In time, and as education becomes the basis of nurse registration, the training for nurses will become clear, focused." Charlotte herself was transitioning, awakening to roles for nurses that would require college education, rather than simple apprenticeship and repetition. For now, she and Annette needed to be accepting and honest with each other, as the teacher and student fluidly moved between roles.

An avid reader, Annette had begun independent study. Given the dearth of textbooks available in the nurses' parlor at the Waltham program, she purchased several books to give herself a background in the discipline. Pulling out Henry Gray's *Anatomy of the Human Body*, or the Doctor's Bible as nicknamed by Alfred, from her green and brown wool carpetbag, Annette turned to the chapter on neurology, focusing on the development of the nervous system. Despite its hundreds of pages of content and detailed illustrations, Annette found it wanting, incomplete without links between normal anatomy and physiology. In time, she thought, perhaps I can rectify this omission with a book of my own.

From the front window at 265 Henry Street, the rainy, bleak, and cold weather was unwelcoming to Lillian's guests, all of whom gathered round the warm fireplace.

Following a hug from Lillian, Annette introduced Charles, who then introduced Alfred and Charlotte. Charles added that they had learned much about Lillian's public health work from Annette. In turn, Lillian asked after Millie and recollected their adventures jumping roofs. Lillian gave a vivid description of the two women, in bloomers and skirts, leaping over a single-foot distance as if it were the Grand Canyon. Laughter and warmth filled the room.

"Lillian, I feel as if I am still in Cambridge," said Charles, smiling at Lillian and shaking her hand. Fall in Massachusetts, he further explained, was consistently inconsistent, with brilliant sunny days highlighting colorful leaves contrasted with dull, dreary days making one yearn for fireplaces.

"Before Jacob arrives, perhaps you can tell us a bit about your settlement." Charles sat down in a straight-backed wooden chair in the first-floor parlor, with other chairs arranged around the fireplace. With a grapevine wreath and tabletop vignette of acorns and gourds decorating the parlor, warmth and fellowship permeated the air. Lillian provided a brief, unassuming summary of her patients, community, and social services work, noting that the building now housed eleven nurses; a janitress, Mrs. McRae; her son, Tommie; and a handyman. She noted that the work of the settlement was generously funded by Jacob Schiff, their benefactor. Although residents were charged either minimally for services or bartered in kind, Lillian indicated that Jacob's support was fundamental to their work.

Concluding her summary, Lillian explained that the laughter emanating from a room adjoining the parlor came from local mothers participating in a home nursing class currently offered by a resident nurse.

"Since we have a few minutes, let me introduce you to the nurse offering the class," said Lillian.

Annette was dumbfounded when Lillian introduced Lavinia Dock as the home nursing class teacher. She only hoped that her face did not reveal astonishment. Tall, slim, erect Lavinia, with hair piled high on head, straightened, a fixed glower on her face, as she shook hands with Charles, then Alfred and Charlotte.

"We met at a meeting of the General Federation of Women's Clubs in Cambridge, before the Chicago World's Fair," said Annette, extending her hand for Lavinia to take, a gesture unacknowledged.

It was clear that she had remembered Annette's provocation at Ellen's home during that late winter meeting of 1893.

Continuing, Annette said that she was surprised to see Lavinia working and living at the settlement.

"I joined Lillian's family here at the settlement. We are a community of women."

Lavinia turned to Charles, telling him of rumors within the society of nurse leaders that Harvard was interested in offering nursing education. Was this true? she asked him directly.

"Yes, we are," Charles said frankly, gesturing to Alfred to continue the conversation.

Lavinia, however, averted her eyes from Alfred, instead saying sharply to Charles, "You cannot offer nurse training. You are not a hospital."

"Correct," replied Charles without hesitation. "We plan to offer nursing education, not apprenticeship training."

"Once nurse legislation is approved in states," she shot back, "nurses will be registered to practice only upon completion of thorough hospital training."

"That, Miss Dock, remains to be seen," Charles replied, just as Jacob Schiff entered the room, escorted by Tommie. Lavinia turned and left the room.

Ignoring the tension and focusing on the moment, Lillian escorted her guests to her office, a smaller room off the parlor, outfitted with a large desk, lamp, paper, and an inkwell and steel point fountain pen. With room for all to sit comfortably, she positioned Jacob, Charles, and herself in front of the desk. Alfred, Annette, and Charlotte sat in a small couch against one wall. Lillian knew that whatever happened next would be of importance long after the settlement drifted into history's fog.

"Charles, I support your school of nursing at Harvard. While we agree that science is the foundation for improved health, science alone will not improve people's lives. It is the nurse in the community that facilitates integration of healthy behaviors. Nurses teach, encourage prevention, care for sick families, and so much more. And so, I pledge to endow a professorship in public health nursing the very day the Massachusetts legislature approves the establishment of a Harvard school of nursing."

Pulling his watch from his vest pocket, Jacob checked the time as Charles, Alfred, Annette, and Charlotte rose to thank him for his support. Seated, Lillian smiled, quietly knowing that her work would endure at Harvard and, perhaps, find its way across the nation.

Before leaving, Jacob addressed Charles directly.

"Remember your roots. In 1869, you cautioned higher education trustees to avoid recklessly spending capital in bricks and mortar. Rather, you advised, spend money and time in identifying the best teachers and administrators. Finding your best people will be your first step in advancing the new school." Pointing to Lillian, then subsequently sweeping his hand toward Alfred, Annette, and Charlotte, Jacob smiled.

"You are beginning with all, and all at their very best. Stay that course." And with a final little bow and smile, he left the office.

Lillian ended the day by leading her visitors to the back of a cooking class, called the *Good Times Club*, taught by a young nurse. Lavinia served as her circulating cooking assistant. For five cents weekly, noisy residents crowded into the class, wedged against a large table to watch the master cook craft nutritious meals. Since many of the Yiddish-speaking residents also wished to learn English, the teacher also served as a language instructor, with a thick Brooklyn accent. Charles was moved by what he witnessed, the joy of learning, of doing, of each woman part of something larger, both greater than and different from, what had come before.

When the class ended, Lavinia left the room quickly, avoiding all farewells. Sampling a spoon of stew from the young nurse while the classmates looked on with delight, Charles did not notice she had left.

The next morning, the crew congratulated themselves on a successful venture as they adjusted themselves in comfortable seats on the New Haven Railroad that would return them to Boston from the Pennsylvania Railroad Station in Jersey City.

"We are truly moving ahead with funding," Charles said. "But I wonder about the differences between Henry Street and Waltham. How will we prepare Harvard graduates for the range of needs that we ourselves have seen?"

Charlotte replied that she was herself struggling to integrate her experiences in the Lower East Side with her own in Waltham. She knew that the curriculum would be key in offering health care to whatever it was that America was, at breakneck speed, becoming.

She noted that the American Society of Superintendents of Training Schools for Nurses had outlined a standard two-year uniform curriculum at their third annual meeting in Philadelphia in February, 1896. A friend of Mary M. Riddle, assistant superintendent of Boston City Hospital, who had attended the meeting, Charlotte had the opportunity recently to review the uniform curriculum, advanced by the Society to secure standardization in methods and subjects, over afternoon tea. She also reported that Mary Adelaide Nutting, superintendent of nursing at Johns Hopkins Training School, gave a summary report of statistics on the hours worked by pupil nurses while on duty, with seventy-three and a half hours per week the average.

Nutting contended that hospitals needed more pupils, less hours worked per week per pupil, and more theoretical instruction, in order—and here Charlotte recalled the phrase—"to avoid graduating weary and spiritless souls only capable of mediocre work." Mary had encouraged Charlotte to attend the fourth annual meeting of the Society to be held in Baltimore in February, 1897, saying that she was eager to hear Nutting, President of the Society, give the welcoming address for the convention.

Given the size of her hospital and training school, Charlotte could participate as a visitor at the next meeting, and subsequently apply as an associate member, according to Mary. Alfred agreed that Charlotte needed to attend the next convention, assuring her that the hospital would cover her expenses. The more she knew about varied curricula, he reasoned, the better for Harvard.

Charlotte, while pleased for her role in Charles's exciting venture, was fatigued. She wished only to close her eyes, enjoy the sun streaming through the train window, and rest. Alfred, proud of Charlotte, sensed her fatigue. He knew that her alliance to plans for nursing at Harvard came at a price. If it was true that the arc of humanity bent toward justice, then Charlotte, he knew, was surely part of the process.

Christmas of 1896 was unlike past holidays. Change, Annette thought, had now become the order of the day. Although Caroline and Amos's home was decorated festively, as in past years, the atmosphere was one of anticipation, an urgency to contribute, to make society more meaningful, always better. A certain restlessness, a drive to ferment, was palpable in the Fiske home.

As guests gathered in Alfred and Elizabeth's home on New Year's Eve, 1896, Annette, previously scheduled for a twelve-hour shift at Waltham Hospital, was worried that the special privilege she received to attend this party might be deemed unfair to her pupil nurse colleagues. Yearning for the security of her quarters on the top floor in the Cutler House, Annette missed her hospital night tour, knowing that she always returned to her standard frame single bed at the end of her shifts feeling satisfied, content that she had helped one or more patients sleep comfortably.

Despite her general unease, Annette was radiant in her evening dress, accompanied by Martin, staying in Philip's old room during the holidays.

Elizabeth and Marguerite provided a musical interlude before dinner featuring Handel's "O Lovely Peace" as guests sampled appetizers including sausage puffed pastries, Scottish potato scones, leeks in cheese sauce with crackers, and bacon-wrapped oysters. Alfred served his guests chilled Sauvignon Blanc to accompany his wife's appetizers, easing them into discussions regarding progress toward the Harvard School of Nursing.

Gathering Alfred, Annette, Millie, Alistair, and Martin to chairs set in a semicircle around the fireplace, Charles requested updates on progress, stating that he would speak to a new topic once their reports were completed. Alfred and Alistair, speaking first, reviewed efforts with Arthur Lyman, Matthew Campbell, and Jacob Schiff. Millie and Annette declared the four-year curriculum complete as draft one, with clinical rotations currently planned by

Alfred. Millie indicated that refinements would perhaps be made following Charlotte's visit to Baltimore.

Charles then introduced what he thought would be an innovation: review by one objective nurse educator. "Is there any nurse leader who might be objective about a Harvard curriculum?" he asked.

"No," replied Annette rather quickly, quiet up to this moment. "However," she continued, "we might be well-served if we consider two ideas. First, invite a highly respected nurse leader to comment on the content of our curriculum, as you suggest, Charles. And second, appoint a current nurse leader to oversee the Harvard effort. Such a nurse leader could report to Alfred, who reports to you."

The president of Harvard, Annette continued, would appear welcoming to outsider comments, magnanimous in sharing Harvard's proposed curriculum. If such a request was rejected, then the crew could anticipate any future objections when the school came before the legislature for approval. And, on what objective basis, Annette theorized, would a nurse leader reject an offer by Harvard University to serve as the lead nurse in designing a new school of nursing? Knowing Annette best, Millie caught a gleam of mischief in her friend's light-blue eyes.

"If you consider these tactics," Annette continued, "then I would suggest, Charles, that you invite Lavinia Dock to serve as both our curriculum reviewer and your lead nurse. If she declines your offer, then we will better understand battles ahead of us." Annette fell quiet as the room considered her plan.

Alfred broke the silence.

"What you propose, Annette, is tricky, although interesting. If Lavinia rejects our requests and explains her rationale, then I agree that we are better armed for our future. Yet if she agrees, we have brought a hungry fox into our fold."

Charles suggested that Alfred write to Lavinia, inviting her to review the curriculum and to serve as nurse leader in planning the Harvard School.

"Lavinia will report to you and hold title at Harvard, and you will report as director directly to me," Charles concluded. He understood the risk and, with Annette, calculated that Dock's loathing of him would stand in the way of whatever better angels were left in her angry soul.

"What of registration and legislation?" asked Charles, looking at Alistair and Martin to conclude the evening's discussion.

Alistair, aware that the American Society for Superintendents of Training Schools for Nurses planned to discuss nurse registration at their annual convention in February of 1897, reported that the team working on the *Riddle Bill* had drafted language for another version of a nurse registration bill. The bill, to be proposed by co-sponsors Joseph Walker, Samuel McCall, and Lewis Apsley, was to be reviewed by Mary Riddle and others in a meeting already scheduled for after the Society's convention. Martin, Joseph Walker, Jr., and David crafted language in the *Riddle Bill* to be similar to that of medicine.

Alistair and Martin realized that nurse leaders, favoring hospitals, would demand specific language in the bill regarding several consecutive years of hospital work. And the corollary, rotations in district nursing or home care, would be decried, considered irrelevant, even barbaric in the burgeoning era of hospital sanitation.

Rallying, Alfred reminded the crew that the Waltham School existed before the hospital, which was founded with the encouragement of nurses who wanted another level of care for very ill residents. He reminded them that he had always welcomed the construction of hospitals, critically important for serious illness, but not at the expense of home and district nursing.

"Hospitals, home care, and district nursing exist together. Pupil nurses need experiences in all such settings." Reason, he believed, would prevail.

Reason supported, Charles thought in silence, by the finances of Lyman, Campbell, and Schiff, and by the alumni who were integrated into the Massachusetts legislature. He realized that so much was due to the efforts of this clever classic scholar, compassionate physician, and those they had gathered around them.

After dinner, they celebrated the New Year, toasting to 1897, a year, claimed Charles, of great strides toward the establishment of the Harvard School of Nursing.

"To nursing!" toasted Charles.

As the party ended, Annette and Martin slipped out to the gazebo and sat in companionable silence.

"Where do you think we'll be when you complete your nursing program?" Martin asked, grasping Annette's hand, as if to will the response he wanted from her.

"We will be here, Martin. Planning our lives together."

Charlotte liked Baltimore. While brutally cold, her journey to attend the nurse superintendents' convention was an adventure she had not anticipated. The convention was held in the Donovan room of the Johns Hopkins University buildings, and Mary Adelaide

Nutting, superintendent of the training school and president of the society, provided the opening address.

"Our day is new," she began, "and the rules and traditions of yesterday do not meet our needs." Numerous and great opportunities for usefulness, Nutting continued, existed in America, particularly for nurses.

Absorbing papers, discussions, and nurse chatter voraciously, Charlotte learned much of nurse leaders' beliefs at the convention.

Nutting, Charlotte learned, had succeeded the founding superintendent of the Johns Hopkins School, Isabel Hampton Robb, who had claimed at a previous convention that a superintendent's duties were first, to the hospital, and second, to the nurses under her. To Charlotte, Robb rooted the society in idolization of hospitals. Charlotte winced at Robb's view of the nurse as "handmaid of that great and beautiful science in whose temple she may only serve in minor parts." As hospital equipment, the nurse was vehicle to hospital growth, as characterized in the American Medical Association's 1869 recommendation. Better work, Robb claimed, and stricter discipline are possible in hospital training schools as compared to work done by hired nurse graduates.

Awash in nurse leaders' language and beliefs, Charlotte now clearly recognized the relationship between hospitals and training schools. Inextricably symbiotic, hospitals needed the bone and sinew of pupil nurses, a phrase she overheard Lucy Drown from Boston say to friends during a break between sessions, in order to operate profitably. And, since Nutting claimed that the ranks of nursing were becoming overcrowded and the quality of nurses inferior, she advocated institution of a uniform curriculum, a longer course of training, and shorter hours of duty. District and home nursing were omitted as curricular reforms. Nutting,

Charlotte understood, advocated nurse registration as a means to alleviating nursing's two evils: overcrowding and inferior quality.

Realizing that her school in Waltham was an anomaly and that nurse leaders were too deeply entrenched in their beliefs to dissuade, Charlotte decided to leave the convention early. If nurse registration were to be linked to years of hospital training, then graduates of the Waltham School would not be registered as the program was currently offered. And a Harvard School of Nursing curriculum would have to include consecutive hospital rotations throughout the program, as well as home and district nursing experiences and college coursework.

I must inform Alfred and Annette, Charlotte thought. These women, she worried, enjoyed oppression.

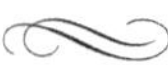

"Alfred, I will appoint you as Professor of Nursing at the next Harvard Corporation meeting," said Charles. "Your appointment is an important step in what will undoubtedly be our successful venture."

"Charles, such a professorship will madden the majority of nursing leaders," replied Alfred, knowing now, with certainty, that the leaders envisioned nursing as a respectable profession only for women.

"All the better. We want to distinguish ourselves from them." Charles congratulated Alfred, asserting that he was the perfect choice.

Alfred had received a letter from Lavinia Dock. It contained her response to his invitation to serve as nursing superintendent of the proposed Harvard School of Nursing.

"Charles, Lavinia has rejected my invitation. In fact, it is a scathing refusal." Passing the letter quickly to Charles, as if very hot to touch, Alfred added that "in her estimation, I am in no way fitted for such a directorship, my chief disqualification evidently being my gender." Continuing, Alfred said she thought him a pest, a pretender, a jealous man in a woman's nursing world.

"This is a complex situation, with nursing tied up in women's movements. It is beyond health care. Beyond hospitals. I feel that there is no bottom to Lavinia's distrust for, indeed hatred of, men." Alfred sighed.

"I agree, Alfred," said Charles, noting silently that Annette's plan had worked. As she had imagined, Dock revealed that she had no reasoned objection to the Harvard School other than blind hatred. And now, Charles realized that he was free to administer the program in nursing as he thought best.

Annette, completing her probationary period at the Waltham School in winter 1897, was eager to engage in district nursing under the supervision of her assistant superintendent. Fully trained in sanitary methods, Annette secretly vowed to avoid invalid cooking, routine housekeeping, and window and floor mopping throughout her career. Home economics, a phrase that became popular in the late 1800s, was viewed broadly by Annette as a human responsibility, one not specific to any particular profession and certainly not integral to nursing.

The Harvard School of Nursing will not offer home economics, pledged Annette.

Annette became immersed in clinical rotations, lectures, and Sunday afternoon discussions among pupil nurses and doctors at the Waltham Hospital. Helping people where they live became her passion. Teaching family members good eating, regular exercise, safe sexual practices, avoidance of alcohol and illegal drugs, smoking cessation, need for vaccinations, and other health behaviors enlivened Annette. Carefully documenting each case, including all health teaching and illness care provided, Annette categorized her summaries according to health care areas important to Alfred, Charlotte, and Lillian.

Her district nursing travels exposed Annette to the poor health status of many Waltham residents. Chief among them were tuberculosis, malnutrition, sexually transmitted infections, pregnancy-related morbidity, and addiction. Jacob Schiff is correct, Annette thought, our new school must focus on public health nursing. She wondered if Lillian would consider accepting an endowed professorship at Harvard? Would she ever leave her beloved East Side?

The transition from district nursing to hospital nursing was dramatic to Annette. Hospital care, she had always believed, was clearly vital to saving the lives of extremely ill patients. Grateful to have bedside experiences with seasoned nurses and doctors, she immediately appreciated the fragility of humans. Managing damage to the human body after prolonged exposure to sustained unhealthy behaviors, such as alcohol intoxication or excessive eating, required herculean efforts. Likewise, trauma, oftentimes resulting from industrial accidents, left patients mutilated, psychologically damaged, and unable to work. Eager to learn and assist, Annette became an invaluable member of the hospital team, one capable of prioritizing patients' needs after a few seconds' assessment.

The more difficult task, Annette realized, was faced in the community. Advocating for healthy behaviors was as difficult as trauma care, without assurance of sustained changes. Additionally, the burden of mental illness seemed, at times to Annette, to be insurmountable. Nursing the five to six mental patients housed in the tenement adjacent to the Cutler House seemed futile. How are such patients managed? What outcomes are expected? How does a nurse prepare to treat such patients?

Faithfully progressing through her clinical rotations, Annette painstakingly adjusted to each setting, receiving accolades from her teachers. Enjoying return demonstrations on living models, she learned the essential skills of bandaging, massaging, bathing, caring for wounds, and the activities of daily living. Over time, Annette accepted the dearth of textbooks available for her additional reading, knowing that the creation of a literature base in nursing would come with time. In her quiet moments, she envisioned herself writing a textbook for nurses on the structure and functions of the body. For now, she and other pupils must simply do it, then subsequently learn to do it better, and finally, to do it well. And then, she hoped, to write it.

Charlotte and Annette became increasingly friendly, with Annette serving as Charlotte's confidante. In the summer of 1897, Charlotte sought Annette's advice about a very unusual situation. She explained that Canadian women hoped to celebrate the sixtieth anniversary of Queen Victoria's accession to the British throne by establishing a general district nursing service in Canada. When Lady Aberdeen, wife of the general counsel, saw that district nursing was taught in America only at the Waltham Training

School, she requested that Charlotte return to Canada to establish district nursing services in her native country.

"Annette, I am both thrilled and frightened. Yes, I would love to return to my country to do this work, but I am also needed here." Charlotte, tears welling in her eyes, handed the letter to Annette.

After reading the letter, Annette advised Charlotte to request a leave of absence for three months to accept the challenge.

"If you leave in January 1898, then you would return in April that same year. Who knows? Perhaps you may wish to relocate to Canada permanently. You are a professional woman. You have opportunities to advance." Pointing to the letter, Annette said that the letter was one such way.

"Annette, if I am asked to name my replacement, I will name you. You are clearly able to do this work, and to serve as a teacher. Would you accept my naming you as my temporary replacement, or perhaps permanent replacement if I remained in Canada?"

Knowing that she was being groomed for a role at the Harvard School of Nursing once established, Annette understood that the Waltham School would close in two years, transitioning to the new baccalaureate program. Annette realized that if she replaced Charlotte as the Waltham superintendent, either temporarily or permanently, her period of service would be relatively short.

Together, they drafted a letter to Alfred, requesting a three-month leave of absence for Charlotte, with Annette as a temporary replacement.

Alfred was not surprised when he received Charlotte's letter of resignation as superintendent effective on July 1, 1898. At that time, managers of the Cutler Home, now deemed inadequate to house the growing number of nurses at the Waltham School, sought a new location for the school. Concurrently, Annette worked with the nurses and doctors at the hospital and school while also planning with Alfred, Millie, and Alistair for the new Harvard School of Nursing.

Amidst a whirlwind of change, Annette graduated for the third time, in June of 1898, from the Waltham Training School for Nurses. She had been a student for two years and its acting superintendent for six months.

Although she had enjoyed her previous graduations from Radcliffe College, Annette felt joyful, fulfilled, and serene as she accepted her diploma from Alfred, along with the school's medal. The medal, a gold medallion, was inscribed with the Latin words *fides* and *spes* — faith and hope. The diploma, considered by the school administrators as an incentive to do good work, was recognized as a lifetime achievement.

At twenty-five, Annette was prepared to contribute. With Martin at her side during the short family party following her graduation, Annette eagerly awaited what would be an evening celebration to be held at Elizabeth Agassiz's home.

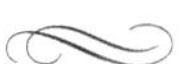

During Annette's graduation ceremony at the Waltham School, Charles, Elizabeth, Jacob, Arthur, Matthew, Alistair, and David sat at the capital statehouse, awaiting the legislature's decision regarding the establishment of a Harvard school of nursing. With faculty, alumni, community leaders, hospital administrators, physicians, and others seated behind the seven main speakers, the stateroom on the groom's side was crowded. On the bride's side of the room, opponents to the Harvard question were few, primarily members of the American Society of Superintendents of Training Schools for Nurses. When asked for their reasons to oppose, the presentations were inconsequential, one quoting a nurse leader as having said at a society meeting that the nurse was a handmaid of the science conducted in hospitals. Another indicated that nurses were hospital equipment who obeyed physicians. Hospitals, opponents claimed, were the only place where nurses could be trained effectively.

After a brief session, the elderly chairman of the hearing observed that legislators, regarding the proposal for a Harvard school of nursing, only dealt with facts, data, and available resources needed to mount the proposal. Rising from his chair and taking off his eyeglasses, he looked directly at the primary spokesperson for the society. He reminded her that the motion under debate was an educational one and that church was separated from state in America. "We do not deal with handmaids, temples, or equipment," he concluded. "That language is fodder of religion."

He then turned to Charles.

"Congratulations, President Eliot. Your request to establish a school of nursing at Harvard University is approved. You have demonstrated the resources, curriculum, clinical sites, and administrative plan to effectively operate a school. You may enroll students in your new school effective academic year 1900–1901."

Once Elizabeth Agassiz welcomed her guests, she offered a preface to her celebration.

"Tonight," she said, "we celebrate the culmination of synchronized work over six years led by Charles. Marked by their glorious differences, his colleagues, disciplined and passionate, succeeded."

Continuing, she noted that with approval of the Harvard School of Nursing, built on the previous establishment of Radcliffe College, women, nursing, and health care could flourish, with positive impact on quality of life of all Americans.

With celebration throughout the house, Annette and Martin slipped out temporarily, walking to Appleton Chapel on the Harvard Campus. Unlocked, the chapel smelled pine-fresh, with a woody aroma infusing a quiet, dimly lit, tranquil building.

"Martin, I did not know that you were religious," Annette whispered.

"I'm not," he said, "but I am in love. In this quiet place, I ask you to marry me."

As Martin reached for a ring in his jacket pocket, she placed her hand over his, holding it fast. She could feel his hand release the box within.

She took his hand in hers, kissed it softly, and set the course for their lives.

"Call me Annie."

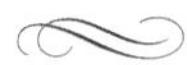

Gesturing to Millie to join him at the dessert table, Charles noted that their work together would begin on Monday. Knowing that Millie had resigned her teaching assistant position at the Cambridge School for Girls now that the academic year had ended, he was eager to assign her a workplan, from recruitment of students to securing of endowments. There was much to do in preparation for the first class of Harvard's School of Nursing.

"How early can you be at my office?" asked Charles, eyebrows arched.

"When the sun rises." Millie smiled.

"Then let's plan our first commencement," said Charles.

He beamed for a moment, then scratched his cheek, adjusted his glasses, and returned to work.

LIFE
Special Report, 1975
Healthy America: A Celebration

A Beginning

"**O**ur US Health System—the USHS—is the envy of the world."

So declared Rear Admiral S. Paul Ehrlich, Jr., Acting Surgeon General. Appointed by President Gerald R. Ford, Ehrlich, wearing his service dress blue uniform, spoke on the occasion of the Harvard University School of Nursing's seventy-fifth convocation in Cambridge, Massachusetts, on Wednesday, September 4th.

"Today, you begin your life in the USHS, a service of your country."

Removing his deep-blue military cap with the insignia of the USHS and date 1920, Ehrlich relaxed his stance as he addressed his audience of baccalaureate, master's, and doctoral students, and their faculty and families.

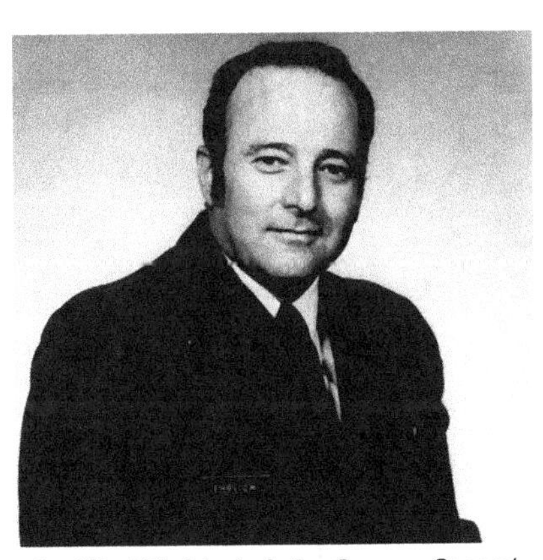

Saul Paul Ehrlich, Jr. Acting Surgeon General, United States Public Health Service, 1973-1977.

"*Exactly what* do other countries envy about our USHS?" Ehrlich asked.

"They envy our focus on health."

"Our comprehensive services."

"Our free health care services."

"Our universal health record system."

"Our coordinated health services."

"Our abandonment of insurance health plans."

"And our soaring life expectancy and skyrocketing health indices."

Informally called the Nation's Doctor, Ehrlich oversees the USHS, a complex enterprise established in 1920 to protect, promote, and advance the health of all citizens.

"The country's shifting focus from disease to health began here, at your school, in 1900. Be proud," Ehrlich advised. "Appreciate events of the past—*your* past. In the US, health is a human right."

The convocation was also the occasion of the posthumous award of the Harvard Medal to Annette Fiske-Byrne, founding dean of the Harvard School of Nursing. Elizabeth Byrne, Annette's daughter, accepted the award on her behalf.

Events in our nation's past, particularly during the period when the Harvard School of Nursing was established in 1900, reveal how the road taken by Fiske-Byrne and her colleagues led to the formation of the USHS.

Conflicting Paths

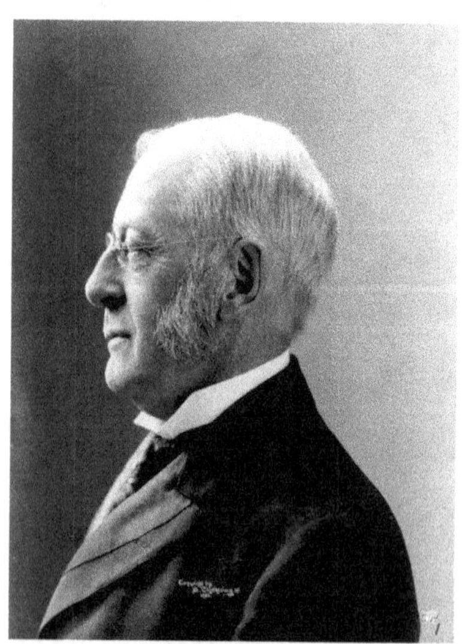

Charles William Eliot (1834 - 1926). President, Harvard University, 1869-1909.

Charles W. Eliot became Harvard's twenty-first president in 1869. The country was ravaged by conflict and far behind Europe in industry and commerce, and Eliot was determined to Harvardize the nation's higher education system, especially through the advancement of science. At first, that city on a hill was to be built by men.

Yet as the suffrage movement gained momentum and women's clubs organized, Elizabeth Agassiz, wife of Harvard zoology professor Louis Agassiz, called on Eliot to provide college education for women. On March 23, 1894, their goal was accomplished when Governor Frederic Greenhalge signed an act of incorporation for Radcliffe

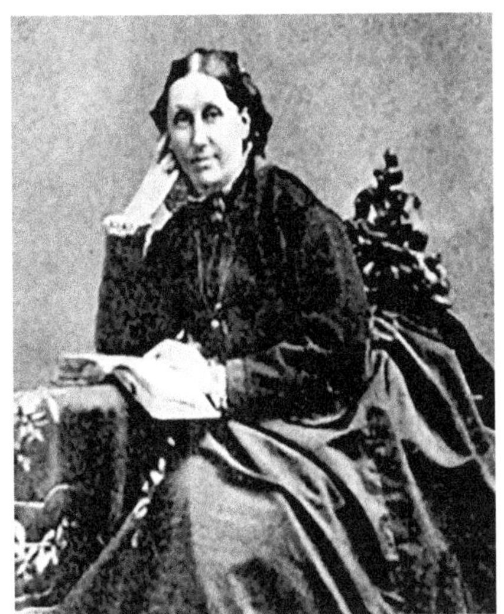

Elizabeth Cabot Agassiz (1822 - 1907). President, Radcliffe College, 1882-1903.

College, authorizing it to confer academic honors and degrees to women. Harvard now had a sister institution.

Calls for equal rights, however, did not end there.

The 1893 Chicago World's Fair had framed the US as the leader of the free world. The professions, especially medicine, nursing, engineering, and education, were organizing. Leaders wished to make everything new, to galvanize power.

During the fair, nurse leaders founded the American Society of Superintendents of Training Schools for Nurses. Seeking to professionalize nursing, society members vowed to change the public's image of a nurse. Embracing a uniform curriculum to standardize training, nurse leaders followed medicine's model of licensure. However, unlike physician registration that linked licensure to graduation from a college or university awarding medical degrees, nurse leaders demanded graduation from a two-year hospital apprenticeship program as prerequisite for licensure.

Hospitals flourished as they established training schools for nurses. Unpaid pupil nurse apprentices provided patient care twenty-four hours a day, seven days a week under sporadic supervision by physicians and nursing superintendents. Additionally, pupils prepared meals, mopped floors, folded laundry, and conducted all other housekeeping functions. Their payment for such services was room and board and a certificate of completion after two years of hospital service.

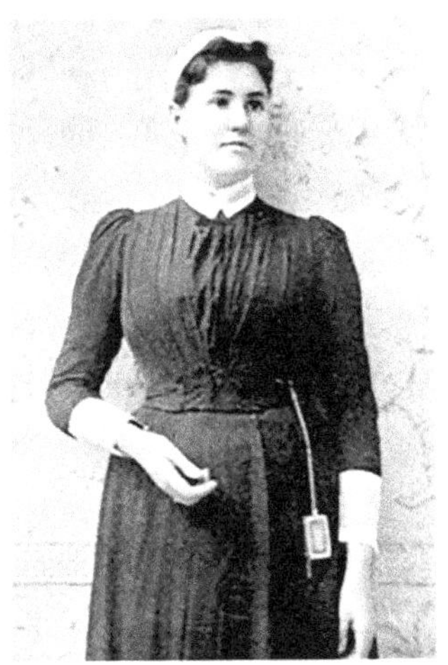

Isabel Hampton Robb (1859 - 1910). Superintendent, Johns Hopkins School of Nursing, 1889-1894.

Nurse leaders idolized hospitals, enthralled with stringent cleanliness and sanitary methods. Identifying pupils as the needed bone and sinew equipment of hospitals, nurse training became inextricably intertwined with hospitals. Nurse leader Isabel Hampton Robb likened nurses to handmaids of hospitals, themselves temples, in which monastic rules of obedience, silence, and loyalty were demanded.

The emphasis on training in hospitals framed a strong anti-educational bias among nurses in the late nineteenth century.

It was the wrong direction for what would soon be called the American Century.

Other forces, and individuals, soon emerged to change everything.

Annette and Alfred

In the nineteenth century, residents of the highly educated, densely knit region known as Back Bay were influential far beyond Massachusetts. Sometimes, with those who know each other well, change occurs after the workday is over.

Eliot and Agassiz often dined together with their faculty, Harvard alumni, and business leaders who lived and worked in this region. As she

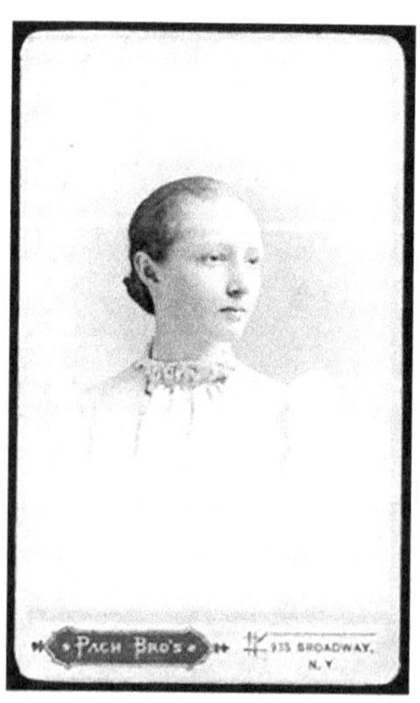

Annette Fiske-Byrne (1873 - 1953).
Radcliffe College, Class of 1891.

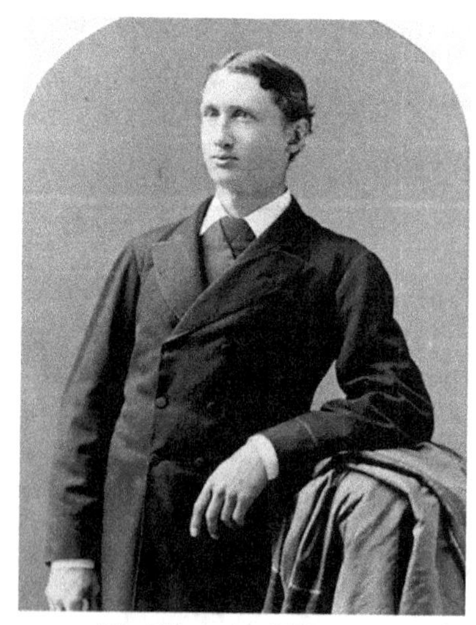

Alfred Worcester (1855 - 1951).
Harvard College, 1878.

did in a recent interview with Daniel Schorr for CBS News, Elizabeth Byrne sometimes tells the story of her mother's first meeting with Alfred Worcester, a Harvard Medical School alumnus and member of the medical staff of Waltham Hospital. At a dinner party with Eliot; Agassiz; Fiske-Byrne's father and mother; and her uncle, Francis J. Child, the Boylston Professor of Rhetoric and Oratory at Harvard, Annette met Alfred. Together, they would put health care on the path celebrated by Admiral Ehrlich at the Harvard convocation.

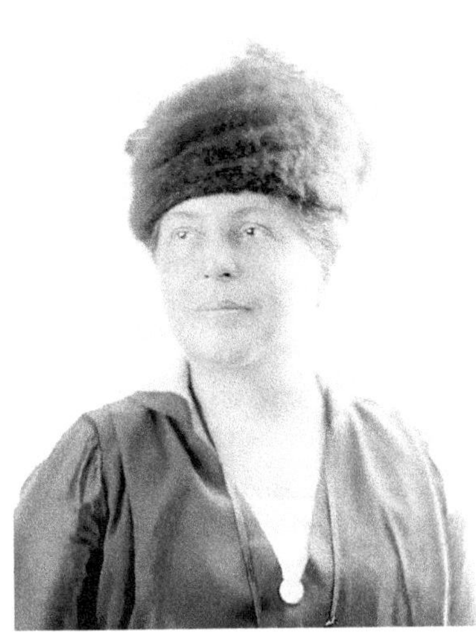

Lillian D. Wald (1867-1940).

Captivated by his descriptions of the work conducted at the Waltham Hospital and Training School, Fiske-Byrne soon toured both the facilities and private homes of patients, beginning her lifelong engagement in nursing. A classics scholar earning her AB and AM degrees in ancient languages from Radcliffe College in 1894 and 1896, she claimed that she had never truly lived until she became a nurse. She graduated from the Waltham School for Nurses in 1898.

According to her daughter, as a pupil nurse, Fiske-Byrne delighted in working at milk stations, the Waltham Watch Factory industrial clinic, immunization centers, and the baby hospital. Her visits to Lillian Wald's Henry Street Settlement in the Lower East Side of Manhattan grounded Annette to the importance of public health. It was at

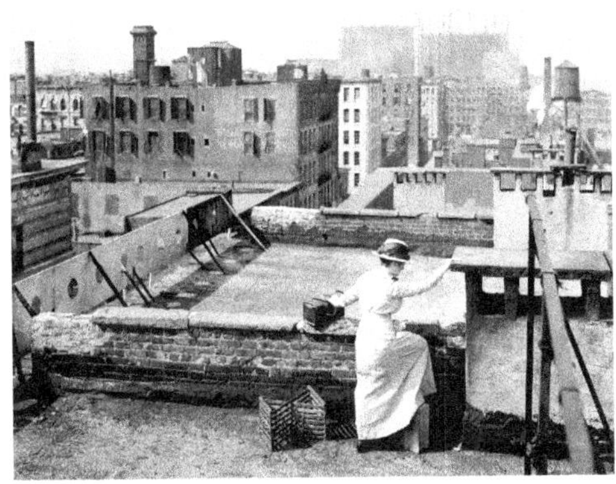

Henry Street Settlement Visiting Nurse. Circa 1918.

the settlement that Annette met Lillian Wald. Alongside Wald, Fiske-Byrne hopped from one rooftop to another in the Lower East Side.

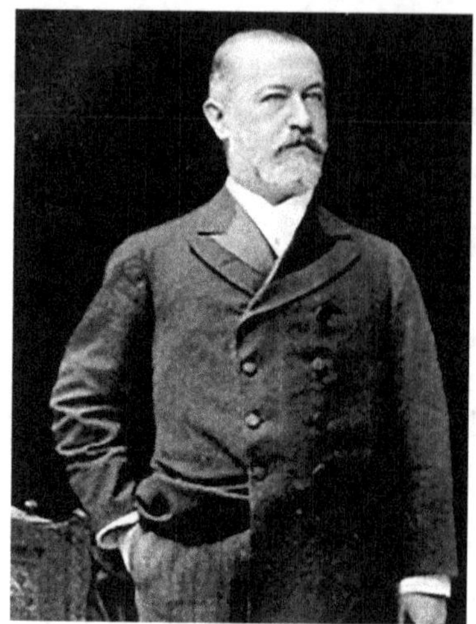

Jacob Schiff (1847 - 1920).

At the settlement, Fiske-Byrne also met Jacob Schiff, a health care financial champion of Wald.

Schiff's focus on public health forever framed Fiske-Byrne's views on nursing.

To Wald, all citizens were entitled to equal, quality health care.

To Schiff, justice could be advanced for citizens through *Tzedakah*, the Jewish principle of charitable giving.

Fiske-Byrne became an advocate for health education, recognizing that hospitals, while extremely valuable for learning acute care, were not the only, or primary, site of practice. She also began to realize that the Society of Superintendents' proposed requirements for nurse licensure were too restrictive in their mandated hospital apprenticeships.

Annette and Alfred, with the support of Eliot, focused on establishing the Harvard School of Nursing, complete with a four-year Harvard baccalaureate nursing degree. Licensure, while critical, was to be a post-school concern.

Their hope was that, with medicine and dentistry, nursing would form a trinitarian view of health care for America.

Endowments and Legislation

A private institution, Harvard has always operated on endowments, and Eliot kept to that tradition. He obtained funding from Matthew Campbell, textile mill owner and member of the Harvard Board of Overseers. He obtained funding from Arthur Lyman, a longtime friend to the Waltham Hospital and School, encouraging him to transition his financial support to Harvard.

And, perhaps most significantly, he obtained funding from Schiff, who had previously gifted Harvard to establish a museum dedicated to the literature, history, and remains of the Semitic peoples. Passionate about public health, particularly for the Jewish community living in the Lower

East Side of Manhattan, Schiff supported the first public health nursing professorship in the new school.

With endowments secured, Charles, Annette, Alfred, and Elizabeth Agassiz—with several key alumni—planned strategies to secure approval for a Harvard school of nursing from the Massachusetts legislature.

Lobbying to secure a board of registration of nurses that would license nurses based on education, Eliot found support from Congressmen Joseph Henry Walker, Lewis Apsley, and Samuel McCall. An act co-sponsored by them to provide for the registration of nurses was approved by the Massachusetts legislature on April 27, 1910, to take effect on October 1, 1910.

Health Triumphant

The Harvard School of Nursing torpedoed the American Society of Superintendents of Training Schools for Nurses. The Society's key objective, establishment of hospital-based, uniform, standardized, apprenticeship nurse training programs, ended as the Harvard model took root.

Hospital administrators were the first to read the tea leaves. They began closing their training schools at the turn of the century.

Nurses, like physicians and dentists, were now considered professionals.

Colleges and universities across the US soon followed Harvard's lead, organizing baccalaureate nursing programs, coordinating clinical education with local hospitals and other facilities. The exponential hospital expansion of the late nineteenth century slowed, as tertiary care became emphasized by specialty physicians employing increasingly sophisticated and complex diagnostics and treatments offered only in acute care hospitals.

With medicine and dentistry, nursing flourished as it carved out primary and secondary prevention efforts through regional, state, district, and community nursing services. An upswing in vaccination rates, coupled with decreased incidences of sexually transmitted infections, became trends in the early twentieth century that continue today. Equally significant, the nation's poor child morbidity and mortality statistics gradually improved, as appropriate childcare was promoted.

As health promotion activities advanced, public health initiatives flourished.

The demand for epidemiological and biostatistical data accelerated rapidly in the first decade of the twentieth century. Combining forces, Fiske-Byrne and Henry Asbury Christian, dean of Harvard Medical School, approached Harvard's new president, A. Lawrence Lowell, to consider a new school, a school of public health. In 1913, this new school was approved, working collaboratively with the nursing, medical, and dental schools on the Harvard campus.

In time, the American Society of Superintendents of Training Schools for Nurses evolved as well, spurred forward by the transition of hospital training schools to degree-granting programs throughout the country. In 1912, the Society reorganized at the National League for Nursing Education. Forty years later, it changed again, becoming what we recognize today: the National League for Nursing, an organization assuming responsibility for accreditation of nursing degree programs throughout the country.

Health and Wealth

By 1920, Congress recognized that health insurance was a costly demand on citizens. Over time, government assistance would be needed by those unable to pay for coverage. With healthy behaviors promoted and practiced, adult lifespan would increase, and morbidity and mortality data would improve. And, while primary and secondary prevention strategies were less costly than tertiary care, steps were needed to ensure no-cost, equal quality care for all. At the same time, World War I illustrated costs of a maldistributed, sporadically delivered health care system.

The USHS emerged as a solution.

With universal, no-cost health care coverage for all citizens paid through taxes, the USHS eliminated individual health insurance plans that had been tied to employment and managed as a trade union benefit.

Consistent evidence-based health policies were needed to keep the USHS operating under current scientific findings. In 1928, Fiske-Byrne and Worcester, supported by the American Nurses Association and the American Medical Association, lobbied Congress to establish a Center for Health Promotion and Disease Prevention. With depression looming throughout the country, Congress agreed to establish the CHPDP, with headquarters located in Massachusetts. Shepherded under the watchful eye of Governor Martin Byrne, Fiske-Byrne's husband, the CHPDP headquartered in Boston on the corner of Beacon and Bowdoin Streets, where it remains today. S. Lillian Clayton, then president of the American Nurses Association, was named as first director of the CHPDP. Soon after its establishment, the CHPDP initiated a Division of Environmental Health, dedicated to basic and applied research exploring the relationship between human and environmental health.

Today

Thanks to the groundbreaking efforts of Fiske-Byrne and Worcester, and the academic leadership of Eliot, the US remains an immigrant gateway to opportunity, to education, and to health. And so it is that the four-story Harvard School of Nursing building on Longwood Avenue has special significance.

Rising to receive her mother's award, Elizabeth Byrne, who had lived the history of the school, stood in front of the brilliant banners, the School of Nursing flag placed centrally above the double front doors. The largest of the crimson, white, and black flags, the nursing flag was majestic, with *veritas* embossed in black letters on images of white pages. The lamp of life, symbolic of nursing, was stitched boldly in black and white below the lettering. On either side of the outside columns, American flags stood tall in sturdy brass stands, each with eagle toppers.

Harvard President Derek Bok presented the award. "Today, we honor Annette Fiske-Byrne for her courage, conviction, and determination to align our country with health promotion."

Byrne, accepting the medal, gave her appreciation of Harvard's recognition of her mother's life work. She said she had been blessed to witness the consequences of that work for subsequent generations. She concluded simply.

"I am grateful. My country is grateful."

So say we all.

Author Afterword

"That a great university like Harvard should open its doors to nurses is magnificent," wrote Sophia Palmer, editor-in-chief of *The American Journal of Nursing*, in an editorial comment in the January 1905 volume.

Palmer then continued, adding a darker note.

"From a broad outlook the whole plan must be most cordially commended by the nursing profession, but from a nearer standpoint we feel somewhat distrustful of the immediate result."

Why distrustful?

In 2007, I discovered Palmer's editorial as I browsed the library stalls at the University of Medicine and Dentistry of New Jersey (UMDNJ) in Newark, New Jersey. Researching information on the history of nursing in the state, I spent much time during my sabbatical reading articles to the right, and to the left, of my search targets. My focus, the confluence of power and politics on the evolution of nursing in New Jersey, led me down unfamiliar stacks of the library and unexpected paths of thought.

The more history I discovered, the more uncomfortable I became. Driving home, I often felt discouraged—and somewhat embarrassed—by the actions and behaviors of past nursing leaders. Evidence of oppression, monastic practices, laborious apprenticeship training, and severely restricted work opportunities after graduation clouded my spirit and hobbled my devotion to write dispassionately. Sioban Nelson's 2003 book *Say Little, Do Much: Nursing, Nuns, and Hospitals in the Nineteenth Century* haunted me.

Historically, nursing did not have a joyous entrée as a profession. Since I had not learned of nursing's history in my undergraduate education, the myopic views of early nurse leaders in the late nineteenth and early twentieth centuries stunned me.

It was a distrust I recognized.

Reading Palmer's editorial, I was awash with memory. As professor and founding dean, I established a school of nursing at UMDNJ (today part of Rutgers, the State University of New Jersey) in the late twentieth century. In that process, I discovered that nurses throughout the state, and many in other states, distrusted my president, my institution, and me. Viewed a pariah wishing to control all of health care education in the state, Stanley S. Bergen, Jr., inaugural president of the university, strategically planned and executed the establishment of schools of medicine, dentistry, nursing, public health, and allied health in his twenty-seven years in office. Each step he took, and each I took with him, was considered as an aggression on turf claimed by others.

Almost a century earlier, Charles W. Eliot, president of Harvard University, had a goal to infuse the nation with competent health care professionals, to Harvardize America with highly educated leaders across diverse fields, including medicine, dentistry, and nursing. As I wrote the book you have just read, I could not help but think of Bergen and Eliot, two goal-oriented men who were extremely focused, strategic, political, and confident.

Yet, while nursing found its origin in Eliot's lifetime, events during his watch framed nursing within a complex anti-educational framework that far too often clouded the profession's growth. Reductionism lingered through Bergen's presidency.

I completed my manuscript, publishing it in 2009 as *On Duty: Power, Politics, and the History of Nursing in New Jersey*. The Harvard proposal, however, continued to haunt me. Shortly after the publication of my book, I visited Harvard University, spending a week in the special collections and archives.

I focused on Alfred Worcester, his reminiscences, correspondence, and other materials. Since Annette Fiske featured in his writings, I also gathered information on her. Having earned her baccalaureate and master's degrees in Greek and Latin, Annette earned her nursing diploma from the Waltham School, eventually becoming a faculty member in that school. Alfred and Annette were a team, working in concert with Eliot. Anti-modern modernists, this trio sought radical contextualization within a growing culture of industrialization, urbanization, and capitalism. The hospitalization of America had begun, as well as Eliot's Harvardization of America. Absent was a Harvard school of nursing. In 2010, I published a paper in *Nursing Inquiry* on what I considered then and now as a catastrophic failure.

While pleased that the article was published, I remained oddly resentful that a Harvard school of nursing had not been established at that time. Professional schools in medicine, dentistry, law, and divinity were founded and had flourished at Harvard. Eliot set expectations for professional education during his presidency, and professions clamored to be in his tent, not out of it. Nursing vehemently demanded to be outside the tent, setting the stage for role confusion for decades into the future.

Since collegiate education was not linked to licensure in the early twentieth century, the registered nurse license has never historically recognized differential scope of practice based on education. Without mandating collegiate education with consequent award of degrees, as occurs in medicine, registered nurse licensure devolved to requiring only completion of an accredited nursing program, including both hospital diploma and degree-granting programs. Thus, a nurse with a hospital diploma is licensed as a registered nurse, as is one with an associate degree, or one with a baccalaureate or graduate degree.

A nurse is a nurse is a nurse.

To this day, I remain enraged. I well know that radical anomalies precipitate change, and the profession I love — the thing in me that goes all the way down — had failed to benefit from what could have been a century's worth of innovation.

In my experience as an academic nursing administrator, the proposal for a school of nursing at the University of Medicine and Dentistry of New Jersey disrupted the nursing community, much as Alfred Worcester, Annette Fiske, and Charles W. Eliot's proposal did at the beginning of the century. Even as the New Jersey nursing community coalesced against my institution's proposal, we focused on our mission, vision, and goals. We strategized. We negotiated and compromised on tactics to achieve success. We sought allies. And we methodically examined the claims of our enemies.

When presenting our proposals to the state for approval, we, like Alfred, Annette, and Charles, faced the bride's and groom's sides at the committee hearing. Our side, the groom's side, was a diverse constituency of educators, businessmen, and health care administrators. The bride's side primarily included nurse educators, nurse organizational leaders, and members of a newly formed New Jersey group called the Partnership for the Advancement of Academic Nursing, or, as I called it, the PAAN Club. Organization, political clout, and planned strategy won the day. Our graduate program began in 1990, the School of Nursing founded in 1992.

I had created, with my colleagues, a disruptive anomaly that resulted, for my nursing colleagues, in chaos. Yet, in time, we witnessed incorporation of change in systems calling for just that. In time, my colleagues and I led efforts for licensure of nurse practitioners in New Jersey, and we witnessed change for many who had been previously underserved. In 2013, I wrote about that in *The Door of Last Resort: Memoirs of a Nurse Practitioner*. While, to this very day, I still feel marginalized in nursing, I have also enjoyed the sheer freedom associated with being an anomaly. I relished the time when there was no one to say no, no one to condemn. Just freedom to think, to create, and to risk. In my role as dean, I took risks. I asked *why not?* rather than the elementalist question of *why?*

Like my imagined Annette, I was fortunate to have been surrounded by supportive, educated, loyal risk-takers. Bergen, Anthony Forrester, David Gibson, and Paul Larson were the crew that built the School of Nursing at the University of Medicine and Dentistry of New Jersey. Like Charles Eliot, Stanley Bergen wanted all at their best. All these years later, that seems a marvelous wish.

And so, in this book, I fulfilled it for Annette.

Frances Ward
Palm Harbor, Florida

Works Cited and Consulted

My historical fiction in *Annette: A Nurse's Story* focuses on nursing education in the late nineteenth century. The novel is embedded in events surrounding the establishment of Radcliffe College, the impact and outcomes of the 1893 Chicago Columbian Exposition, the founding of the American Society of Superintendents of Training Schools for Nurses, the development of women's organizations, the suffrage movement, and the eventual establishment of the Harvard University School of Nursing. Key characters include Charles W. Eliot, president of Harvard University; Annette Fiske, a nurse and scholar of Latin and Greek languages; and Alfred Worcester, a physician. Each is quite real, but the events featured in the novel are imagined paths that, were they to have occurred, would have produced the culture of health described in the fictitious *Life* magazine article I wrote to conclude the book. The following resources were valuable to understand the social, cultural, political, and public health environment in which the novel takes place.

Annual reports for first (1894), second (1895), third (1896), and fourth (1897) Annual Conventions of the American Society of Superintendents of Training Schools for Nurses. National League for Nursing Collection, Barbara Bates Center for The Study of The History of Nursing, University of Pennsylvania. Web.

Billings, John Shaw, and Henry Mills Hurd, eds. *Hospitals, Dispensaries and Nursing; Papers and Discussions in the International Congress of Charities, Correction and Philanthropy, Section III, Chicago, June 12th to 17th, 1893.* Baltimore, Maryland: Johns Hopkins Press, 1894. Web.

Billings, John Shaw, and Henry Mills Hurd. "Section Four
     on the Hospital Care of the Sick, the Training of
     Nurses, Dispensary Work, and First Aid to the Injured.
     *The International Congress of Charities, Correction, and
     Philanthropy*, June 12-18, 1893." *Hospital* 13, no. 331 (January
     28, 1893): 290.

Burgess, John. "Francis James Child: Brief Life of a Victorian
     Enthusiast: 1825 – 1896." *Harvard Magazine*, May-June,
     2006. Web.

Carnegie, Andrew. "Wealth." *North American Review* CXLVII,
     June 1889. Rpt. *The Gospel of Wealth and Other Timely Essays*,
     Edward C. Kirkland, ed. Cambridge, Massachusetts:
     Harvard University Press, 1962. Web.

Chapin, Charles V. *The Sources and Modes of Infection*. New York:
     John Wiley and Sons, Inc., 1910. Web.

Cooper, Glen M. "Swedenborg, Emanuel." In *Encyclopedia
     Britannica*. Web.

Croly, Jane Cunningham. *The History of the Women's Club
     Movement in America*. New York: H. G. Allen and
     Company, 1898. Web.

Dickens, Charles. *Bleak House*. London: Penguin Classics, 2003.
     First published 1853.

Dickinson, Emily (Published anonymously). "Nobody Knows
     This Little Rose." *The Springfield Daily Republican*, August 2,
     1858. Web.

Dock, Lavinia Lloyd. *Hygiene and Morality: A Manual for Nurses
     and Others, Giving an Outline of the Medical, Social, and Legal
     Aspects of the Venereal Diseases*. New York: G. P. Putnam's

Sons, 1910. Web.

Dock, Lavinia Lloyd. *Text-book of Materia Medica for Nurses*. New York: G. P. Putnam's Sons, 1890. Web.

Eliot, Charles W. *A Turning Point in Higher Education: The Inaugural Address of Charles William Eliot as President of Harvard College, October 19, 1869*. Cambridge, Massachusetts: Harvard University Press, 1869. Web.

"Eliot, Charles W. (1834-1926)." Harvard Square Library. Web.

Eliot, Charles W. "The New Education." *The Atlantic* 23 (February 1869): 203-20. Web.

Eliot, Charles W. "The New Education Part Two." *The Atlantic* 23 (March 1869): 358-67. Web.

Ellis, Havelock. *The Nationalization of Health*. London: T. Fisher Unwin, 1892. Web.

Fiske, Amos Kidder. *Beyond the Bourn: Reports of a Traveler Returned from the Undiscovered Country*. New York: Fords, Howard, and Hulbert, 1891. Web.

Fiske, Annette. *Structure and Functions of the Body: A Hand-book of Anatomy and Physiology for Nurses and Others Desiring a Practical Knowledge of the Subject*. New York: Wentworth Press, 1911. Web.

Fiske, Annette. *First Fifty Years of the Waltham Training School for Nurses*. Boston: Harvard Medical School Alumni Bulletin, 1949.

Forrester, David Anthony, ed. *Nursing's Greatest Leaders: A History of Activism*. New York: Springer Publishing Company, 2016.

Galton, Francis. *Inquiries into Human Faculty and its Development.* New York: Macmillan and Co., 1883. Web.

Garofalo, Mary E., and Elizabeth Fee. "Lavinia Dock (1858 – 1956): Picketing, Parading, and Protesting." *American Journal of Public Health* 105, no. 2 (February 2015): 276-77.

Gay, Peter. *Modernism: The Lure of Heresy.* New York: W. W. Norton & Company, 2008.

Gordon, Anna Adams. *The Beautiful Life of Frances E. Willard.* Chicago: Woman's Temperance Publishing Association, 1898. Web.

Hampton, Isabel Adams. *Nursing: Its Principles and Practice for Hospital and Private Use.* Baltimore, Maryland: Press of John H. Williams Company, 1893. Web.

"Harvard College: Inauguration of Charles W. Eliot as President." *New York Times,* October 20, 1869 Web.

Harvard Dental School. *Annual Announcement of the Dental School of Harvard University for the Year 1891-1892.* Cambridge: Harvard University Press, 1891. Web.

Harvard School of Dental Medicine. "About HSDM." The President and Fellows of Harvard College. Web.

Harvard Medical School. "About HMS." The President and Fellows of Harvard College. Web.

Harvey, David. *The Condition of Postmodernity: An Inquiry into the Origins of Cultural Change.* Cambridge, Massachusetts: Basil Blackwell Publishing, 1989.

Hippocrates. *Oath.* Commentary by Francis Adams. Volume 1. London: Sydenham Society, 1849. Web

Hippocrates. *Oath*. Translated by Francis Adams. Volume 2. New York: William Wood and Company, 1886. Web.

Hippocrates. *On Airs, Waters, Places*. Translated by Francis Adams. Volume 2. New York: William Wood and Company, 1849. Web.

International Congress of Charities, Correction and Philanthropy. *Report of the Proceedings of the International Congress of Charities, Correction and Philanthropy*. Baltimore: The Johns Hopkins Press, 1894. Web.

James, Edward T, Janet Wilson James, and Paul S. Boyer, eds. *Notable American Women: 1607–1950: A Biographical Dictionary*, Volume 1. Boston: Belknap Press of Harvard University Press, 1971.

James, Henry. *Charles W. Eliot: President of Harvard University, 1869 – 1909*. (2 vols.). Boston, Massachusetts: Houghton Mifflin, 1930. Web.

Johnson, Thomas H., ed. *The Complete Poems of Emily Dickinson*. Cambridge, Massachusetts: The Belknap Press of Harvard University Press, 1951.

Keller, Helen. *The Story of My Life: An Autobiography*. Mineola, New York: Dover Publications, 1996.

Marcus, Alan I., and Howard P. Segal, eds. *Technology in America: A Brief History*. London: Palgrave Macmillan Publishers, 2018.

McCord, David. *An Acre for Education: Being Notes on the History of Radcliffe College*. Cambridge, Massachusetts: Crimson Printing Company, 1958.

Morison, Samuel Eliot, ed. *The Development of Harvard University*

Since the Inauguration of President Eliot 1869-1929.
Cambridge, Massachusetts: Harvard University Press,
1930.

Morison, Samuel Eliot. *Three Centuries of Harvard 1636 – 1936.*
Cambridge, Massachusetts: Harvard University Press,
1946.

Nelson, Sioban. *Say Little, So Much: Nursing, Nuns, and Hospitals
in the Nineteenth Century.* Philadelphia, Pennsylvania:
University of Pennsylvania Press, 2003.

Nightingale, Florence. *Notes on Nursing: What It Is, and What It Is
Not.* New York: D. Appleton and Company, 1860. Web.

Nutting, Adelaide Mary, and Lavinia Lloyd Dock. *A History of
Nursing; The Evolution of Nursing Schools.* New York: G. P.
Putnam's Sons, 1907.

*One Hundred and Eleventh Annual Catalogue of the Medical School
of Harvard University 1893 – 1894.* Cambridge: Harvard
University Press, 1893.

"Our history." Henry Street Settlement. Web.

Peabody, Francis Greenwood. *The Problem of Charity: An
Introductory Address to the International Congress of Charities,
Correction and Philanthropy 1893.* London: The British
Library of Political and Economic Science. Web.

Pich, Hollie. "Various, Beautiful, and Terrible: The Life and
Legacy of Ida B. Wells-Barnett." *Australasian Journal of
American Studies* 34, no. 2 (December 2015): 59-74.

Radcliffe College. *Circular of Information, 1896.* Cambridge,
Massachusetts: Radcliffe College, 1896. Web.

Radcliffe College. *Circular of Information, 1897*. Cambridge, Massachusetts: Radcliffe College, 1897. Web.

Report of the Proceedings of the International Congress of Charities, Correction and Philanthropy. Baltimore: The Johns Hopkins Press, 1894. Web.

Richards, Linda. *Reminiscences of Linda Richards: America's First Trained Nurse*. Boston: Whitcomb and Barrows, 1915. Web.

Riis, Jacob A. *How the Other Half Lives: Studies Among the Tenements of New York*. Mansfield Centre, CT: Martino Fine Books, 2015. First published 1890. Web.

Robinson, Lelia Josephine. *HistoryLink.org*. Web.

Roca, Julius. "Inventing an Ethical Tradition: A Brief History of the Hippocratic Oath." *Legal Ethics* 11, no. 1 (2008): 23-40. https://doi.org/10.1080/1460728X.2008.11423898

Rosen, George. *A History of Public Health*. Baltimore: Johns Hopkins University Press, 2015.

Sedgwick, William T. *Principles of Sanitary Science and the Public Health*. New York: The Macmillan Company, 1914. First published 1902. Web.

Starr, Paul. *The Social Transformation of American Medicine: The Rise of a Sovereign Profession and the Making of a Vast Industry*. (2nd ed.). New York: Basic Books, 2017.

Swedenborg, Emanuel. *Heaven and Its Wonders and Hell from Things Heard and Seen*. New York: Swedenborg Foundation, 1946. First published 1758. Web.

Swedenborg, Emanuel. *The True Christian Religion Containing the Universal Theology of the New Church*. New York: Swedenborg Foundation, 1946. First published 1771. Web.

The Society for the Collegiate Instruction of Women. *Announcement Fifteenth Year 1893-1894*. Cambridge, Massachusetts: W. H. Wheeler, Printer, 1893. Web.

Turner, Alexander Paul. *Plain Directions for the Care of the Sick, and Recipes for Sick People*. New York: Mutual Life Insurance Company of New York, 1875. Web.

Wald, Lillian. *The House on Henry Street*. New York: Henry Holt and Company, 1915. Web.

Waltham Training School for Nurses 1885 – 1921. Waltham, Massachusetts. Web.

Ward, Frances. *Door of Last Resort: Memoirs of a Nurse Practitioner*. New Brunswick, New Jersey: Rutgers University Press, 2013.

Ward, Frances. *On Duty: Power, Politics, and the History of Nursing in New Jersey*. New Brunswick, New Jersey: Rutgers University Press, 2009.

Ward, Frances. "A Road Not Taken: The Proposal for a Harvard School of Nursing." *Nursing Inquiry* 17, no. 2 (June 2010): 128-141.

Weeks, Clara S. *A Textbook of Nursing: For the Use of Training Schools, Families, and Private Students*. New York: D. Appleton and Company, 1888. Web.

Wells, Ida Bell. "The Life and Legacy of Ida B. Wells." *The University of Chicago Library*. Web.

Wells, Ida Bell, Frederick Douglass, Irvine Garland Penn, and Ferdinand L. Barnett. *The Reason Why the Colored American is Not in the World's Columbian Exposition*. Chicago: University of Illinois Press, 1999. First published 1893. Web.

Wikipedia Entries: American Woman Suffrage Association; Agassiz, Elizabeth Cabot; Child, Francis James; Dock, Lavinia Lloyd; Fall, Anna Christy; Fiske, Amos Kidder; General Federation of Women's Clubs; Gilman, Arthur; Robinson, Lelia Josephine; Swedenborg, Emanuel; Willard, Frances E.; Worcester, Alfred.

Worcester, Alfred. *Monthly Nursing*. Boston, Massachusetts: D. W. Mason, 1886. Web.

Worcester, Alfred. *Nurses for Our Neighbors*. Boston, Massachusetts: Houghton Mifflin Company, 1914. Web.

Worcester, Alfred. *Reminiscences of Alfred Worcester 1938*. Cambridge, Massachusetts: Harvard University, Countway Library of Medicine, Center for the History of Medicine, Papers, Worcester, Alfred GA95.20.

Worcester, Alfred. *Training Schools for Nurses in Small Cities*. Boston, Massachusetts: Massachusetts Board of Managers, World's Fair, 1893. Web.

Images

(In order of appearance)

Cover. Annette Fiske (1873-1953). Radcliffe College, Class of
1894. Courtesy of Schlesinger Library, Harvard Radcliffe
Institute. http://id.lib.harvard.edu/via/olvwork347267/
catalog

Saul Paul Ehrlich, Jr. (1932-2005). Acting Surgeon General,
United States Public Health Service, 1973-1977. Image
in public domain: https://upload.wikimedia.org/
wikipedia/commons/3/3a/Rear_Admiral_S._Paul_
Ehrlich%2C_Jr.jpg

Charles William Eliot (1834-1926). President, Harvard
University, 1869-1909. Image in public domain: https://
upload.wikimedia.org/wikipedia/commons/0/03/
Charles_W._Eliot_cph.3a02149.jpg

Elizabeth Cabot Agassiz (1822-1907). President, Radcliffe
College, 1882-1903. Image in public domain: https://
upload.wikimedia.org/wikipedia/commons/7/75/
Elizabeth_Cary_Agassiz_portrait.jpg

Isabel Hampton Robb (1859-1910). Superintendent, Johns
Hopkins School of Nursing, 1889-1894. Image in
public domain: https://cwrc.ca/islandora/object/
cwrc%3A10f5eb54-3246-4c60-b818-3395c2e10087

Annette Fiske (1873-1953). Radcliffe College, Class of 1894. Courtesy of Schlesinger Library, Harvard Radcliffe Institute. http://id.lib.harvard.edu/via/olvwork347197/catalog

Alfred Worcester (1855-1951). Harvard College, 1878. Image in public domain: https://upload.wikimedia.org/wikipedia/commons/5/5d/Alfred_Worcester_ca_1878.jpg

Lillian D. Wald (1867-1940). Image in public domain: https://upload.wikimedia.org/wikipedia/commons/5/59/Lillian-Wald.jpg

Henry Street Settlement Visiting Nurse Climbing Over Rooftops. 1918. Photographer Jessie Tarbox Beals. Courtesy of Visiting Nurse Service of New York - Health. High Resolution Image Courtesy of Columbia University Medical Center Library Archives and Special Collections. https://www.henrystreet.org/news/latest-news/sleepless-nights-in-1918-lillian-wald-

Jacob Schiff (1847-1920). Image in public domain: https://upload.wikimedia.org/wikipedia/commons/3/35/Portrait_of_Jacob_Schiff.jpg

ABOUT THE AUTHOR

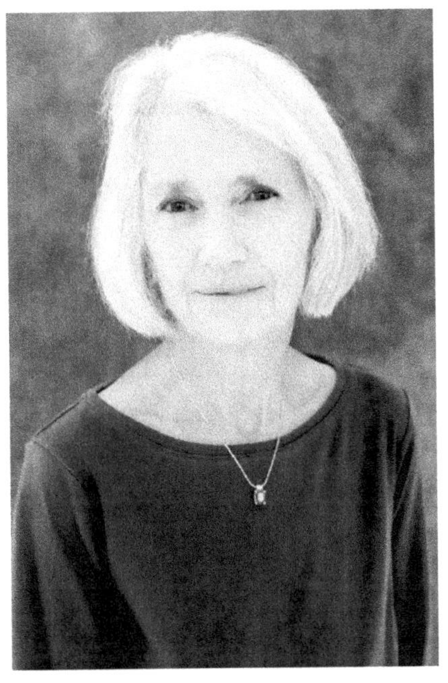

FRANCES WARD, PhD, RN, NP, is Professor Emerita at Temple University, where she held the David R. Devereaux Chair of Nursing until her retirement. Subsequently, she served as executive director of the Pennsylvania Action Coalition, a statewide initiative to improve health care through nursing. She is also the Founding Dean of the School of Nursing at the University of Medicine and Dentistry of New Jersey (now Rutgers – The State University of New Jersey). Throughout her academic and research career, she maintained a clinical practice serving residents in Newark, Camden, and Philadelphia. In 2020 she retired from the profession. *Annette: A Nurse's Story* is her second novel.

9 798876 964151